Making Sense of Practice Finance

Second Edition

JOHN DEAN

with a forewo[rd]
JOHN CHIS[...]

RADCLIFFE M[EDICAL PRESS]
OXFORD and [...]

© 1994 Radcliffe Medical Press Ltd
18 Marcham Road, Abingdon, Oxon, OX14 1AA, UK

Radcliffe Medical Press, Inc.
141 Fifth Avenue, New York, NY 10010, USA

Reprinted 1995

British Library Cataloguing in Publication Data

A catalogue record for this book is available from the British Library.

ISBN 1 870905 94 6

Typeset by Advance Typesetting, Oxford
Printed and bound in Great Britain by Biddles Ltd, Guildford and King's Lynn

Contents

Biographical Note

JOHN DEAN is an accountant who has specialized in the financial taxation and accountancy affairs of members of the medical profession for 20 years. He is accepted as a leading authority on the subject.

John is in considerable demand as a lecturer to doctors and dentists, GP trainees, practice managers and accountants. He also writes extensively for medical and dental journals and his articles can be seen frequently in *Money Pulse*, *Financial Pulse*, *Doctor*, *Medical Business* and other journals.

Making Sense of Practice Finance was his first book; the first edition was published in 1990. *Practice Finance: your questions answered* was published in 1992.

John recently resigned from a long standing position as Director of Medical Services with a national firm of chartered accountants in order to set up his own business, 'John Dean Associates', which offers a full accounting and management service to GP clients. He will continue with his speaking and publishing engagements.

Foreword to the Second Edition

General practitioners, as independent contractors, are responsible not only for the clinical care they provide to patients, but also for the organization and finances of their practices. Young doctors entering general practice may have been attracted by the variety of patients, the prospects for continuing care and the practice of whole person medicine, but they soon discover that they must also acquire the administration skills needed to run a small business with a substantial annual turnover. Without those skills, they will fail the patients they seek to serve and the staff they employ; and they will fail also to maximize their income.

Recent developments in general practice, including the 1990 contract and the introduction of fundholding, have emphasized the importance of value for money and increased the need for organizational and financial discipline. This book is intended to meet that need. It should be essential reading for every GP; and will also be useful for practice managers, practice accountants and vocational trainees.

John Dean and the other contributors to *Making Sense of Practice Finance* are all experts in their fields, and John is renowned as one of the leading authorities in the highly specialized and complex area of general practice taxation and accountancy. The first edition of this book proved to be a vital reference document, and this considerably expanded and updated new edition will, I am sure, prove even more valuable.

JOHN CHISHOLM
Joint Deputy Chairman and Negotiator
General Medical Services Committee
British Medical Association

Making Sense of Practice Finance

Contributors

DAVID BEXON, *Trustee Savings Bank plc*

BOB BOWLES, *Founder Chairman of the Financial Special Interest Group of the Primary Health Care Specialist Group, British Computer Society*

BARRIE BROWN, *Provincial Secretary, British Medical Association*

JOHN CHISHOLM, *Joint Deputy Chairman and Negotiator, General Medical Services Committee, British Medical Association*

MALCOLM DALLEY, *Managing Director, Seabrook Investment Services Ltd*

NORMAN ELLIS, *Under Secretary, Contractor Services Division, British Medical Association*

JON FORD, *Economic Research Unit, British Medical Association*

NICK GILD, *Solicitor*

DOUGLAS SHIELDS, *Medical and Dental Retirement Advisory Service*

Editor

JOHN DEAN, *Specialist Medical Accountant and Independent Adviser on GP Finance*

The Business Side of General Practice

Preface to the Second Edition

THE success of the first edition of *Making Sense of Practice Finance*, published in October 1990, demonstrated a tremendous thirst for knowledge of GPs about their finances. This is understandable; however well trained GPs are in clinical matters, in the early stages of their careers they may nevertheless find themselves struggling to cope as partners with responsibility for turnovers running into many hundreds of thousands of pounds. The practice with a turnover exceeding £1 000 000, which three or four years ago was exceptional, is now becoming relatively commonplace.

All this means that GPs, although delegating much of their management and administrative function to practice managers and other highly qualified staff, must nevertheless remain aware of the manner in which they are paid, how their income is calculated and, in particular, the numerous financial problems arising in partnerships.

Since the publication of the first edition of this book, there have been numerous changes to the manner in which GPs' finances are organized. The 1990 GP contract is no longer 'new'; it is now more than three years old. We are in the third wave of GP fundholding, with undoubtedly more waves to come. Every effort has been made to include up-to-date information available on current trends in practice finance, and to highlight ways in which GPs can organize their affairs to their long term benefit.

In a book of this size, it is clearly not possible to cover all the financial regulations which affect the often unusual manner in which GPs' finances are organized. However, the major points have been addressed, and the GP who finds that these are not applicable to his own position is advised to consult specialist advisers for an informed opinion.

For the sake of brevity and to avoid the use of contorted English, it has been assumed throughout that all GPs are male, and all practice managers female. Although this is clearly not the case, readers are invited to convert this to their own situations as necessary. Any references to the finances of individual practices, or doctors, are purely for example and bear no relation to any known practices. This particularly applies to the specimen accounts set out in Chapter 18, whose purpose is solely to provide points of reference for explanations of accounting procedures in this and other chapters.

The preparation of this book would not have been possible without the assistance of contributors and specialist colleagues, who have helped both by making contributions and reviewing the content at its various stages.

Without them the book would not have been completed. I should particularly like to thank Douglas Shields for reviewing the chapters on pensions and retirement, Jackie Roberts for her assistance with the chapter on fundholding, and Kate Irving for her valuable comments at the review stage.

JOHN DEAN
August 1993

Since the publication of the second edition in December 1993, there have been a number of far-seeing changes in the world of GP finance. In particular, the pending introduction of the current year basis of tax assessment, together with self-assessment procedures, will be dealt with fully in future editions.

In late 1994 it was announced that the VAT self-supply scheme, which has for some years applied to the development of GP surgeries, would end with effect from 1 March 1995.

On 29 November 1994, in the Chancellor's Budget, it was further announced that, effectively, amendments will be made to the 'de-minimis' rule, which will make it highly unlikely that any GP will be qualified to register under this scheme. In particular, Chapter 45 should be read with this in mind.

Apart from this, changes have been made in Appendices A, B and C in order to show new rates of fees and allowances, income tax and insurance levels for 1994/95 and 1995/96.

JOHN DEAN
January 1995

List of Abbreviations

AA	Automobile Association
BMA	British Medical Association
BPA	Basic Practice Allowance
CGT	Capital Gains Tax
DHA	District Health Authority
DoH	Department of Health
DSS	Department of Social Security
EEC	European Economic Community
FHSA	Family Health Services Authority
FIMBRA	Financial Intermediaries, Managers and Brokers Regulatory Association
FSAVC	Free-Standing Additional Voluntary Contribution
GMP	General Medical Practice
GMSC	General Medical Services Committee (of the BMA)
GP	General Medical Practitioner (in the NHS)
IHT	Inheritance Tax
LMC	Local Medical Committee
MMR	Mumps, Measles and Rubella
NHSPS	NHS Pension Scheme
NIC	National Insurance Contributions
PAYE	Pay-as-you-Earn Tax
PGEA	Postgraduate Education Allowance
RCGP	Royal College of General Practitioners
RHA	Regional Health Authority
SFA	Statement of Fees and Allowances (the Red Book)
SMP	Statutory Maternity Pay
SSP	Statutory Sick Pay
VAT	Value Added Tax

1 General Practice Finance Since 1948

The beginning

BEFORE the introduction of the National Health Service (NHS) in 1948, general practitioners (GPs) received their income from two principal sources, private practice and the national health insurance scheme. The estimated net income from these sources was the starting point from which the Spens Committee recommended appropriate remuneration for GPs under the fledgling NHS. Its recommendations, reported in April 1946 but couched in pre-war prices, were referred first to a working party charged with determining distribution and second to an adjudicator (Mr Justice Danckwerts) for revaluation to current prices. The outcome of these two processes is sometimes regarded as having established the principles underlying the financing of general practice as we now know it. However, the report of the Royal Commission on Doctors' and Dentists' Remuneration in 1960 related, for the first time, the average intended net income for GPs for general medical services work as a separate item. Previously, average intended net income had included not only income from other sources but also the Exchequer's share of superannuation contributions.

The Danckwerts adjudication set average intended net income at £2222 per annum for 1950/51 and also recommended a retrospective level of £2055 per annum for the preceding two years. Arrears covering all three years were paid in 1952/53. These figures are, however, not compatible with the current definition of intended net income. After adjustment, they are equivalent to £1975 and £1825 respectively. These net incomes, together with a provision for practice expenses, Exchequer superannuation contributions and income from other sources, represented the Central Pool of remuneration for GPs, a fixed sum whose distribution was based on capitation payments. Prior to the changes introduced as a result of the Family Doctor Charter over the period 1965–7, pure capitation payments accounted for 67% of total gross income, and a system of loadings, also capitation-based, accounted for a further 16%. These have been changed further and radically as a result of the 1990 GP contract (*see* Chapter 19).

A charter for the family doctor service

The Family Doctor Charter, proposed in 1965, is the foundation stone of modern general practice finance. The consequences of the remuneration system it created were dramatic. As well as substantially increasing real net income, the contract changes introduced over the period 1966–7 provided for improvements in the financing of both premises and supporting staff. With respect to premises, an independent corporation was proposed to provide funds for the erection of new purpose-built premises and the modernization of existing ones. This corporation, the General Practice Finance Corporation (GPFC), was set up in 1967. It continued in that form until its acquisition by Norwich Union in 1989.

The 1966 contract also introduced a direct reimbursement system for premises expenditure, which provided incentives for GPs to provide services in a cost-effective manner, embracing economies of scale. Similarly, the introduction of direct reimbursements for the bulk of ancillary staff costs encouraged the development of practice teams. The 1990 contract subsequently recognized that services could be delivered more effectively with smaller average lists.

The net income of general practitioners since 1948

The bulk of the real growth in general medical services (GMS) expenditure since the beginning of the NHS has been accounted for by indirect refunds of expenses. After adjustment for inflation, the net income of GPs has on average increased more slowly and has been subject to dramatic fluctuations over the last 40 years. The retrospective application of the Danckwerts adjudication implies an average intended net income for GPs of £1825 in 1948/49 on a basis consistent with the present. Average intended net income in 1993/94 at £40 610 represents £2273 when expressed in 1948/49 prices. This increase of 25% in real terms is very modest in comparison with increases in gross payments. At present, however, GPs' net incomes are at their highest level since the inception of the NHS and now exceed the previous peak in the early 1970s. Movements in intended average NHS net income since 1948 are set out in Figure 1.1. Many GPs also derive a relatively high level of additional income from sources outside the NHS (see Chapter 9).

Since 1990

With the introduction of the 1990 contract, NHS general practice finance is now a combination of an extension of recent trends and a return to past

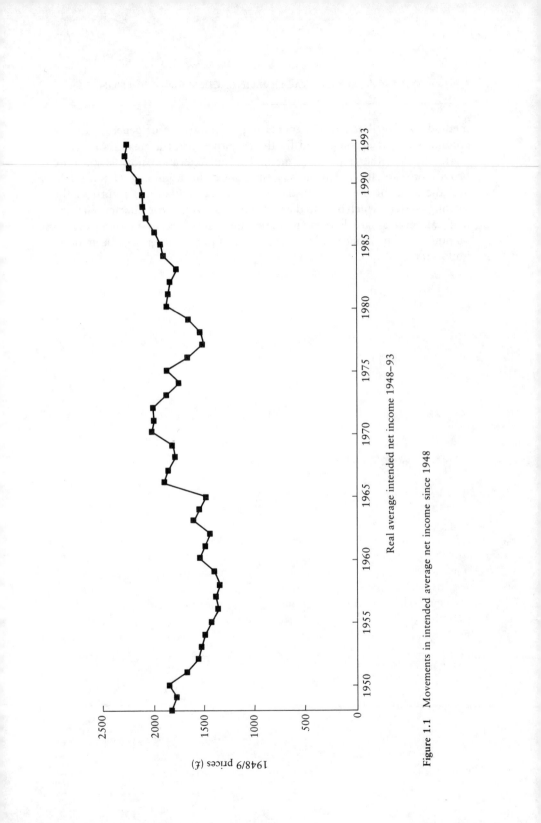

Figure 1.1 Movements in intended average net income since 1948

methods of distribution. The increasing capitalization of general practice continues and is accompanied by the employment of a greater variety of staff. On the other hand, the method of remuneration now leans more heavily on capitation than at any time since the beginning of the NHS, and the form of the new capitation-based system marks a return to the loadings system which operated prior to the Family Doctor Charter. General medical services are becoming increasingly complex to provide and to administer. An understanding of practice finance never has been more important.

2 Independent Contractor Status

An independent contractor is a self-employed person who has entered into a contract of services with another party. This contract for services is fundamentally different from a contract of service that governs employee – employer relationships. A key test, often used to distinguish between these two types of contract, relates to the question of 'control'. Generally, the more control A exercises over B's work, the more likely A is to be the employer and B the employee. Thus, if A can tell B not only what job to do but how it is to be done, A has sufficient control to be B's employer.

However, if the exercise of control is much more diffuse, such that the person doing the work is not told how to do it, the contract is for services and the relationship is between what is confusingly known in legal terminology as 'the principal party' and an independent contractor. Obviously, this test is crude and there are borderline cases, but the status of the NHS GP as an independent contractor has not been seriously questioned in the past. As an independent contractor a GP should not be told by the Family Health Services Authority (FHSA) or Health Board how to practise. FHSAs and Health Boards should seek to persuade and advise, not to direct or control.

The character of UK general practice has been strongly influenced by the independent contractor status of its practitioners. The remuneration system, the organization of practices into partnerships, together with the medico-political institutions that enable GPs to exercise professional self-government, demonstrate this influence.

As independent contractors, GPs exercise discretion and freedom in how they run their practices. This autonomy carries with it the administrative and financial responsibility for running the business itself and also responsibility for the clinical services provided. These responsibilities include providing premises, staff and equipment. If GPs were health authority employees (like hospital consultants), the authority would be responsible for providing these resources.

The main advantages of an independent contractor service are flexibility and adaptability, and the fact that it can offer a more personalized model of care. It also provides opportunities for innovation and diversity without interference, and gives patients scope for choice. Disadvantages may be apparent if the standards of service are allowed to vary widely; those who are responsible for administering GPs' contracts sometimes see this arrangement as untidy and unsatisfactory, because the means of control available to the employer are lacking.

No other health service occupation (apart from the other Family Health Services contractor professions—dentists, chemists and opticians) has this unique partnership with the state, or with the public. In current parlance, general practice is the original 'privatized' sector of the NHS. GPs in other Western developed economies, together with most other professionals, such as dentists, lawyers, architects, surveyors and accountants, are also independent contractors. In the UK, GPs have jealously guarded independent contractor status ever since Lloyd George's national insurance scheme was introduced in 1911. The profession supported the idea of a state-funded medical scheme, but it was adamantly opposed to a salaried service; it recognized that the loss of independent contractor status would undermine the freedom of doctors to practise without state interference and ultimately put patient care at risk. GPs feared that government would seek to direct them in their day-to-day treatment of patients. This commitment to the independent contractor status underlies the policy of the Conference of Representatives of Local Medical Committees (LMCs).

The present arrangements specify precisely the services GPs are required to provide for patients. The terms of service make clear that health promotion and illness prevention fall within the definition of general medical services (GMS). The services that are required of the GP are spelled out in some detail, specifying which procedures should be undertaken and which patients should be offered certain services.

During the debate surrounding the imposition of the 1990 contract, the question was raised as to whether the new Regulations and terms of service were incompatible with the GP's status as an independent contractor. Whilst there can be no doubt that greater control will now be exercised over the work of the GP, both the Government and the General Medical Services Committee (GMSC) of the British Medical Association (BMA) are agreed that the GP should continue to work as an independent contractor. Indeed, in a joint statement from the Department of Health (DoH) and the GMSC, the Secretary of State for Health 'confirmed that the independent contractor status of GPs would not be affected'.

However, the question of whether GPs are independent contractors is not something which can be resolved according to the wishes of the two parties directly concerned. It ultimately depends upon whether the control exercised by FHSAs is sufficiently diffuse to justify retention of the independent contractor status. In spite of the increased accountability required under the 1990 contract and the increased powers of the FHSA, there should be no doubt that GPs continue to work as independent contractors. The old contract also contained detailed specification of certain clinical tasks (such as those relating to the provision of maternity care) and these have never been regarded as incompatible with the independent contractor status.

3 How General Practitioners' Pay is Determined

THE Doctors' and Dentists' Review Body was set up in 1960, as a consequence of the recommendations of a Royal Commission known as the Pilkington Commission. Its remit is to recommend to the Prime Minister the levels of remuneration of doctors (and dentists) working in the NHS.

The Pilkington Commission was concerned to ensure that doctors' pay should not be used as a means of regulating pay movements in the economy; it wanted to see their pay removed from the political arena. The Commission considered various options, including direct negotiations, collective bargaining through Whitley machinery (as used by most health service employees), and arbitration. It recommended an independent review body and laid down the ground rules by which it should operate (*see* Box 3.1).

Box 3.1: Ground rules of the Review Body

1 The Review Body's main task is the exercise of 'good judgement'.
2 Although the Government has the ultimate power to decide, Review Body recommendations must only very rarely (and for most obviously compelling reasons) be rejected by Government.
3 Government should deal with Review Body recommendations promptly.
4 The remuneration of doctors should be determined primarily, although not exclusively, by external comparison with other professionals and similarly qualified employees.
5 Doctors should not be used by Government as part of its machinery for regulating the economy; they have a right to be treated fairly and the profession should assist the Review Body by willingly providing information about their earnings.
6 Doctors' earnings should not be determined according to short-term considerations of supply and demand.

How the Review Body system works

The Review Body is willing to receive evidence from any interested party, but in practice it concentrates on evidence from a few key sources (*see* Box 3.2).

In spite of the increased accountability required under the 1990 contract and the increased powers of FHSAs, there should be no doubt that GPs continue to work as independent contractors. The old contract too contained detailed specification of certain clinical tasks (such as those relating to the provision of maternity care) and these have never been regarded as incompatible with the independent contractor status.

Box 3.2: Principal sources of evidence to the Review Body

1 Written evidence from the medical profession, prepared by the BMA (and from the dental profession).
2 Written evidence from the DoH.
3 Joint written evidence agreed between the profession and the DoH, usually dealing with matters which have been agreed in negotiation.
4 Jointly agreed statistical information, for example evidence on GPs' earnings and expenses.
5 Independent evidence prepared by the Review Body's Secretariat, the Office of Manpower Economics, for example various surveys conducted at the request of the Review Body.

The professions and the Departments of Health (DoH) normally submit their written evidence to the Review Body on the same day and also exchange documents. This means that each party has prepared its evidence 'in the dark' without sight of the other evidence.

The next stage involves oral hearings. The Review Body meets each side and uses the occasion as an opportunity to seek clarification of any subject raised in the written evidence or to discuss other points of concern. The parties will also use the oral hearing as an opportunity to emphasize or update any matter in their written evidence.

Having considered all the evidence, the Review Body reports in confidence to the Prime Minister. Further time usually elapses before the Prime Minister publishes the report and announces a decision on the recommendations.

General practitioners' remuneration

GPs, as independent contractors, are paid a gross income by the NHS, out of which they meet their practice expenses, including such items as staff salaries, the cost of providing surgery premises and motoring expenses. The GPs' payment system is based on a principle known as 'cost plus'; the payments they receive are intended both to cover their expenses and provide a net income.

The Review Body recommends what it considers to be an appropriate level of net income for GPs and, taking account of this recommendation, the Government decides upon the average level of income of all GPs. In fact, individual GPs receive greatly varying amounts depending upon the particular circumstances of their practices—expenses and list sizes differ and GPs provide a varying range of services—so it is rare to find a GP whose earnings precisely coincide with the average figure.

To this net income must be added the component for expenses. All expenses incurred by GPs in providing GMS are paid back to the profession in full: some are paid directly to the individual GP who incurs them (these are known as directly reimbursed expenses); the remainder are reimbursed indirectly on an average basis through fees and allowances. Thus, the amount an individual GP receives in indirectly reimbursed expenses will not necessarily equal expenditure, and in practice there will be a strong incentive for GPs to economize in respect of their own practice expenses (see Figure 3.1).

Although this system of dealing with GPs' expenses is complicated and may lead to anomalies and inequalities, it does recognize the independent contractor status of the GP, which is fundamentally different from that of salaried colleagues employed elsewhere in the NHS. One possible alternative would have been to require each GP to submit to the FHSA a monthly or quarterly claim for expenses, which the FHSA would check (and no doubt question on occasion). If this arrangement had been adopted, the profession would have given up its independence to choose how to run its practices. The significance of this point is not always recognized by those who call for increased direct reimbursement.

It has been argued that, because most practice expenses are repaid indirectly through fees and allowances irrespective of what is spent, the less an individual GP spends on the practice the greater will be his profits. Although there is some truth in this view, it does not represent the whole picture. GPs are directly reimbursed for the cost of many of the most expensive items (for example, surgery premises and practice staff). Moreover, a GP who chooses to underfund his practice will find it lagging behind other practices in the services it can offer; it will not be as attractive to new patients and patients currently on the list may opt to transfer to other practices in the neighbourhood. A contrary and more positive view needs to be put forward.

If those GPs who are unwilling to invest in their practices would overcome their reticence, the profession as a whole would benefit through the indirect

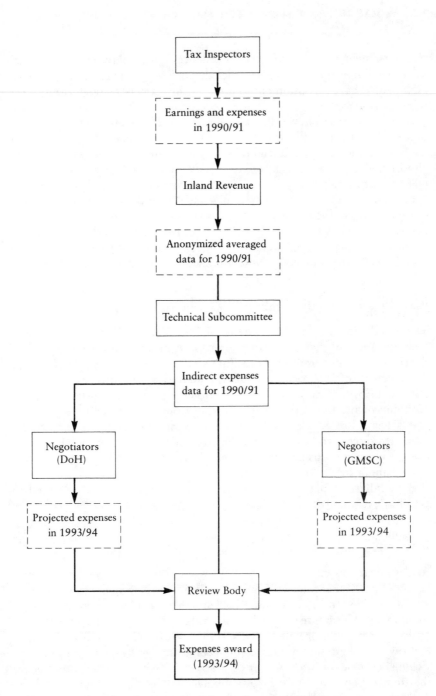

Figure 3.1 Flow chart for expenses mechanism for year 1993/94

reimbursement system and general practice would become more capital intensive. For example, if every GP decided to invest in an ECG machine, the NHS would have no option but to fund this investment through the indirect reimbursement scheme.

An explanation of how GPs' expenditure on defence body subscriptions is indirectly reimbursed illustrates this point. Almost every GP subscribes to a medical defence body, and traditionally the amount each GP pays has been almost the same. These subscriptions have been paid since the establishment of a new GP remuneration structure in the 1960s and therefore the expenditure is built into the system. Defence body subscriptions include those relating to the employment of assistants and locums (although those acting on the GP's behalf should also have their own cover) and payments made under the doctors' retainer scheme. Subscriptions have increased rapidly, yet they can usually be reimbursed at close to the prevailing rate.

Partially and directly reimbursed expenditure

The introduction of cash limits on the funds available to FHSAs for the direct reimbursement of the salaries of practice staff means that the percentage of the salary refunded in respect of future staff appointments may differ from the fixed rate of 70% reimbursement, paid under the former ancillary staff scheme. FHSAs can now exercise discretion in determining the level of direct reimbursement, and in theory it may vary from 0–100%.

A scheme for the partial direct reimbursement of computing costs has been introduced, and provides for the direct payment of a proportion of the costs of purchase, leasing, upgrading and maintenance of a computer system (*see* Chapter 20).

Both fully and partially directly reimbursed expenses are described in detail in Chapter 10.

Indirectly reimbursed expenditure

As described above, each year the Review Body estimates, on the basis of a survey of practice accounts submitted to the Inland Revenue, how much GPs as a body will spend on providing GMS and then calculates an average figure for each GP. This figure is added to the level of pre-tax pay which the Review Body considers appropriate for GPs to earn, known as net intended remuneration, and the resulting aggregate becomes the gross remuneration. The various fees and allowances that comprise a GP's pay are then adjusted so that during the year they yield for the average GP the total gross and net remuneration which the Review Body has deemed appropriate.

This exercise is complex and because the 'targets' set by the Review Body are not always met, any under- or over-payment is allowed for in subsequent years. As the DoH is apprised of how much has been paid to GPs after the end of a financial year, it is not difficult to compare the level of average gross pay received with the original target. Average net pay is more difficult to calculate because this depends upon an analysis of practice accounts.

In order to obtain tax relief, GPs inform the Inland Revenue of the expenditure they have incurred in providing GMS. This is a principal and vital source of information for estimating GP expenses. The Inland Revenue provides each year information (made anonymous) relating to a sample of GPs' accounts. It includes all personal, professional and partnership expenses.

	1992/93 £	1993/94 £	% increase
Gross intended remuneration	59 977	62 303	3.9
Indirect expenses element	20 000	22 190	10.9
	39 977	40 113	0.3
Prior years' adjustments	33	497	
Net intended remuneration	40 010	40 610	1.5

The indirect expenses element represents 35.6% of gross intended income in 1993/94, compared with 33.3% in 1992/93.

Figure 3.2   GPs' intended average remuneration, 1992/93 and 1993/94

General practitioner accounts

As the level of expenses to be reimbursed is always based upon samples of practice accounts submitted to the Inland Revenue for agreement, it is vital that every GP show all the expenses incurred in providing GMS in his practice or partnership accounts and personal expenses claims (*see* Chapters 16 and 41).

Continuous review

The technical subcommittee keeps the system under continuous review. Areas of GP finance currently being reviewed include:

- the effects of the accounting year-end (*see* page 92)
- GP fundholding (*see* Chapter 34)
- the treatment of direct reimbursements (*see* Chapter 10).

4 Fees and Allowances

FEES and allowances currently payable to GPs are set out in the Statement of Fees and Allowances (SFA) which is prepared in accordance with the NHS Regulations containing the GP's terms of service; it may be regarded as a part of the terms of service.

Basic practice allowance (BPA)

A GP only qualifies for the BPA if he has a list of at least 400 patients. This may be an individual list in the case of a single-handed GP or the partnership average list.

Provided a GP has a personal list or average partnership list of at least 400 patients, he will receive a BPA that reflects the list size up to a maximum of 1200 patients.

The level of payment varies so that GPs with smaller average lists receive proportionately more BPA for their patients than those with larger average lists. A lump sum is paid for the first 400 patients, and additional capitation payments are then made for each patient between 400 and 600, 600 and 800, 800 and 1000, and 1000 and 1200. By weighting the level of these payments towards lower list sizes, the BPA is intended to reflect the proportionately greater level of standing expenses of a small practice than of a large one.

Further weighting of the BPA is provided for part-time GPs: a half-time GP's BPA will be significantly more than half of a full-time GP's BPA (*see* Chapter 37).

Associate allowance

Single-handed GPs practising in very isolated areas (eg the Highlands and Islands) are eligible for the associate allowance. This enables GPs in these areas to employ a (shared) associated GP who is able to maintain services for patients during their absence for social and professional purposes.

Deprivation payments

GPs providing services to deprived areas are paid a supplement to the BPA in respect of all patients on their lists who live in areas categorized as 'deprived' according to the Jarman index of deprivation. Each patient living in a deprived area will attract a BPA supplement. GPs with individual or average partnership lists of less than 400 patients, and therefore not in receipt of a BPA, still qualify for deprivation payments for all patients on their list living in deprived areas.

The deprivation capitation payment is paid at three levels according to the degree of deprivation (as measured by the Jarman index) of the area in which the patient lives.

Seniority payments

A seniority payment is made to every GP eligible for the BPA:

1 a first level payment to a GP who has been registered for 11 years or more and has been providing GMS for at least seven years
2 a second level payment to a GP who has been registered for 18 years or more and has been providing GMS for at least 14 years
3 a third level payment to a GP who has been registered for 25 years or more and has been providing GMS for at least 21 years.

Pro rata payments are made to part-time GPs and full-time GPs not eligible for the maximum rate of the BPA. Each job-sharer is assessed for the seniority payment on an individual basis and the level of payment is reduced pro rata according to the hours of availability notified to the FHSA.

Capitation fees

The standard capitation fees continue to be paid at three rates according to the patient's age: under 65 years, 65–74 years and 75 years and over. The level of the fee for patients aged 75 years and over is significantly higher to reflect the new services GPs are required under their terms of service to provide for these patients.

Registration fee

An additional capitation fee is available for all new registrations (except for patients under five years old) to GPs who carry out certain specified procedures in respect of these patients. These procedures should be carried out within three months of the patient joining the list.

Child health surveillance fee

Any GP who wishes to be paid for providing this service must apply to the FHSA to be included in the Child Health Surveillance List. To be admitted by the FHSA on to the List, the GP needs to demonstrate that he is suitably trained and experienced, in accordance with the criteria set out in the Regulations. A capitation supplement is paid for each child patient under the age of five to whom a GP provides developmental surveillance. The child must be registered with the GP for this purpose.

Postgraduate education allowance (PGEA)

This allowance is paid to any GP or associate practitioner who maintains a balanced programme of continuing education. The allowance includes an element to pay course fees and travel and subsistence costs.

To claim the PGEA, GPs are required to submit evidence to their FHSA (or Health Board) that they have attended an average of five days' training a year over the past five years. Although a GP may vary the amount of time spent on courses from year to year, he is expected to achieve a reasonable balance between years.

Courses are divided into three broad areas: health promotion and prevention of illness, disease management and service management. It is necessary to have attended at least two courses under each of these three headings over the five years preceding the claim.

Lunchtime or evening sessions, which offer many training opportunities for GPs (currently regarded as a third of a day), can be accredited as a course if they constitute a planned series of such sessions.

GPs should submit a claim each year to the FHSA (or Health Board) including details of courses attended over the previous five years. If the required criteria (ie 25 days' training and at least two courses in each of the three categories) are met, then the FHSA pays a full PGEA in quarterly instalments.

Single-handed GPs in receipt of rural practice payments are eligible to claim a locum allowance to provide cover whilst attending postgraduate education courses.

Item of service fees

There is no other single heading of income on which a GP's profitability level depends as much as on the efficient claiming of item of service fees. These are, in total, intended to account for 16% of a GP's income. The 1991–2 returned averages for England and Wales showed that the average fees per patient amounted to £4.30.

Many practices achieve higher rates, usually as a result of a busy location; for instance, one would expect practices in holiday resorts to have a much higher than average incidence of temporary resident fees, whereas those in rural backwaters are likely to have below average returns from maternity and family planning fees. Taken as a whole, the average is nevertheless a useful means of judging the financial efficiency of a practice and can act as a stimulus for generating higher levels of income than may previously have been possible. Further details of statistics of this nature are set out in Chapter 19.

Item of service fees are paid for:

- night visits
- maternity medical services (MMS)
- emergency treatment and immediately necessary treatment
- contraceptive services
- temporary residents
- adult vaccinations and immunizations
- anaesthetization or arrest of dental haemorrhage
- minor surgery (*see* Chapter 5).

Night visits

A GP is paid a fee for each visit requested and made between the hours of 10 pm and 8 am to a patient who is:

1 on his list of patients, *or*
2 a temporary resident, *or*
3 a woman for whom he has undertaken to provide MMS, provided the visit is related to these.

A fee is also paid if the GP provides treatment (eg minor surgery) in the surgery in the patient's interests. If care is given in a treatment room of a GP hospital, the fee is paid only if the GP is not on duty or on call for the hospital at the time and the request for the treatment has not come from the hospital. However, if the GP visits the patient in a hospital to provide MMS, a night visit fee is paid if he holds an appointment at the hospital, but was not on duty at the time, or if he does not hold such an appointment in respect of MMS.

A higher fee is payable if:

- the GP with whom the patient is registered makes the visit personally, or
- the visit is made by a partner or another GP from the group practice, or
- the visit is made by an assistant employed by a member of the partnership or group, or
- the visit is made by a regular locum or deputy employed by the partnership or group, provided the FHSA has been previously notified of the employment, or
- the visit is made by a trainee GP employed by the partnership or group, or
- the GP is single-handed or in a group practice or partnership, and is part of a local non-commercial rota which includes GPs outside the group or partnership who have agreed to provide out-of-hours cover for each other; they may also be single-handed or working in a group, but their number must not exceed 10. The FHSA needs to be informed of the details of these arrangements.

In all other cases, a lower fee is payable to the GP with whom the patient requiring the visit is registered.

Maternity medical services (MMS)

A full MMS fee is paid to GPs who provide a comprehensive service during the pregnancy of a patient, including the confinement and postnatal period. In addition, a full postnatal examination at or about six weeks after confinement, and in any event no later than 12 weeks afterwards, must be carried out. The full fee is payable provided that the GP accepts his patient's application to receive these services, and that the application is accepted no less than six weeks before the date of confinement.

The higher rate MMS fee is paid only to GPs included on the Obstetric List.

The full criteria for payment under this scheme are set out in paragraph 31 of the SFA.

Emergency treatment

When a GP on the medical list of an FHSA is called upon, through accident or emergency, to treat a person neither on his own list nor on that of a partner, a fee should be paid for this emergency treatment. The detailed arrangements for payment of such fees are set out in paragraph 33 of the SFA.

Contraceptive services

An annual fee is payable under this heading if a GP accepts a patient, gives advice, and undertakes examinations and prescribes drugs or other aids as necessary. The fee is also payable if the GP takes steps to determine the patient's choice and accepts responsibility for any necessary after-care treatment. An intrauterine device fee is payable for services given in the 12 months commencing from the date of application to fit such a device.

Detailed conditions for payment of fees for contraceptive services are set out in paragraph 29 of the SFA.

Temporary residents

If a GP treats a patient resident in the area on a temporary basis, who is not on his own list, a fee will be paid: at a lower level if the patient expects to remain in the district for 15 days or less; or at a higher level if the patient expects to remain in the district for more than 15 days. In order to be considered as a temporary resident for this purpose, the patient must remain in the area for more than 24 hours. Separate regulations apply with regard to persons resident in holiday camps.

Detailed arrangements for payment of this fee are set out in paragraph 32 of the SFA.

Adult vaccinations and immunizations

Fees are payable for adult vaccinations or immunizations (or any ineligible for target payments) provided the patient is on the GP's own list or that of his partner, or is eligible for treatment as a temporary resident.

Target payments are made for childhood immunizations and pre-school boosters (*see* Chapter 7).

The regulations for payment of fees are complex as they are for treatment given to safeguard against certain conditions on an opportunistic basis. Full details are set out in paragraph 27 of the SFA.

Anaesthetization/dental haemorrhage arrest

In certain circumstances GPs may be called upon to act as anaesthetists or to arrest a dental haemorrhage. Whilst in many practices this will occur infrequently, GPs should be aware of the relevant fees. Detailed arrangements are set out in paragraphs 34 and 35 of the SFA.

Claiming the correct fees and allowances

The NHS GPs' remuneration system is said to be the most complex in the world. It takes several hundred pages of the Regulations and the SFA to define with precision how a GP should be paid. Every practice should ensure that it is claiming the correct fees and allowances; otherwise it will lose out on its remuneration. On the other hand, no claim must be made, whether knowingly or unknowingly, for a fee or allowance to which a GP or practice is not eligible. A false or improper claim can lead to very serious consequences; FHSAs have not hesitated to instigate criminal prosecutions against GPs who have made such claims.

5 Minor Surgery

To claim a fee for this work, a GP must be included in the FHSA's Minor Surgery List. It is paid for minor surgery sessions provided for his or her own patients or those of partners or group members.

No more than three payments can be made to a GP in the same quarter, except that, if the GP is in a partnership or group practice, more payments may be claimed provided that the total number paid in any quarter does not exceed three times the number of partners or members of the group on the medical list on the first day of that quarter.

What is a session?

A session consists of five surgical procedures; they may be performed either in a single clinic or on separate occasions during the same quarter. Procedures will count towards a session if they meet the following criteria:

they are included in this list:

Injections	intra articular
	peri articular
	varicose veins
	haemorrhoids
Aspirations	joints
	cysts
	bursae
	hydrocele
Incisions	abscesses
	cysts
	thrombosed piles
Excisions	sebaceous cysts
	lipomata
	skin lesions for histology
	intradermal naevi, papillomata, dermatofibromata and similar conditions
	warts
	removal of toe nails (partial and complete)

| Curette cautery and cryocautery | warts and verrucae
other skin lesions, eg molluscum contagiosum |
| Other | removal of foreign bodies
nasal cautery |

- they are performed by a doctor on the FHSA's Minor Surgery List
- any other person assisting in a procedure is suitably trained or experienced for the task.

Minor surgery list

A doctor who wants to perform minor surgery should apply to the FHSA for inclusion on the Minor Surgery List. The qualifying criteria are specified in the Regulations.

How to claim payment

Claims should be made on form FP/MS which records basic information about the patient's doctor, the doctor carrying out the procedure and the date and type of procedure. FHSAs check the validity of claims.

6 Health Promotion Payments

FOR many years, GPs have been involved in opportunistic health promotion, planned call and recall of patients for preventive care and the planned management of patients with chronic diseases. Until 1990, this work was undertaken as part of general medical services, without any specific payment or any additional funding; the profession was rewarded within average net remuneration.

However, the GP contract introduced on 1 April 1990 made health promotion a specific obligation under GPs' terms of service. GPs were obliged to give 'advice, where appropriate, to a patient in connection with the patient's general health, and in particular about the significance of diet, exercise, the use of tobacco, the consumption of alcohol and the misuse of drugs or solvents', as well as to offer 'consultations and, where appropriate, physical examinations for the purpose of . . . reducing the risk of disease or injury'.

In addition, GPs were able to claim fees for health promotion clinics. Well-person clinics, anti-smoking clinics, clinics for alcohol control, dietary advice, exercise counselling, stress management, heart disease prevention, and the care of patients with diabetes or asthma generally qualified for payment, and other clinics could also be submitted for approval by FHSAs. So long as the purpose of and arrangements for clinics were approved by the FHSA, there was no limit on the number of clinics for which GPs could claim.

A rapid growth in expenditure on clinics resulted: in 1990–1, £50 million was paid to GPs in Great Britain by way of health promotion clinic fees, in the second year of the scheme £73 million was paid out, and in the third year £80 million was claimed. Although collectively GPs were doing more and more work for the same total pool of money, individual GPs sought to maximize their own income by undertaking increasing numbers of clinics, and the level of activity only stopped climbing with the imposition of a moratorium on 1 July 1992. If a moratorium had not been imposed, there was every reason to suppose that the amount GPs were earning from health promotion clinics would have gone on increasing, with the result that GPs would have been paid less and less for the rest of their work. Indeed, the growth in health promotion clinics was a major factor in the destabilization of the GP remuneration system which occurred after the introduction of the 1990 contract.

This clinic activity was very unevenly distributed among practices, with no activity being recorded in many and substantial amounts in others. The distribution could not easily be explained by the needs of patients, and the problem was undoubtedly compounded by the application of differing approval criteria by different FHSAs and Health Boards. The profession collectively said that it felt cheapened and demoralized by, and cynical about, the operation of the clinic system, coupled with GPs' obligation under the Regulations introduced in 1990 to offer a consultation to patients between the ages of 16 and 75 years who had not been seen in general practice within the preceding three years. There was thus considerable pressure for change in the contractual arrangements governing health promotion, and protracted negotiations were undertaken in order to achieve a new system, and to supersede the requirement for GPs to invite non-attenders for three-yearly checks.

The intention was to fashion a system with greater accountability, greater equitability and greater scientific validity, as well as greater professional freedom, recognizing in particular the value of opportunistic intervention. Both Government and profession wanted to see resources targeted on proven activities which would be of greatest benefit to patients. The negotiations took place within the framework set up by the White Paper *The Health of the Nation*, published in July 1992, and the equivalent Scottish and Welsh strategic guidance, and it was decided to focus health promotion activity on the prevention of coronary heart disease and stroke.

It was also seen that health promotion activities had to be appropriate to local needs and circumstances, and to reflect dialogue between FHSAs, LMCs and GPs. FHSAs and DHAs would need to make information available to practices on other relevant local health promotion activities, so that unnecessary duplication could be avoided.

The payment arrangements would need to encourage the wider availability to patients of consistent health promotion programmes, to produce a more equitable distribution of income to GPs, and to deliver a more predictable year-on-year allocation of resources to health promotion activities. It was therefore decided during the negotiating process that health promotion and chronic disease management should be paid for from a pool within a pool: within the total amount of money available for GPs' remuneration, a fixed sum should be set aside for these activities. The size of that pool was to be similar to the amount spent on clinics during the third year of their operation. Such an approach had the virtues of stopping further devaluation of the amount GPs were paid for the rest of their work (including the treatment of sick patients), of circumscribing the level of total health promotion activity, and of making it easier to resist the inclusion of additional activities in the work of GPs without the provision of new money to pay for them. Additionally, the risk of overpayments being made to the profession—which would then need to be clawed back under the Review Body's balancing arrangements (*see* Chapter 3)—would be controlled by a system of annual bidding and fee adjustment.

Transitional arrangements and priorities reflecting local circumstances

Despite the concentration of the care programme on coronary heart disease, stroke, asthma and diabetes, and despite the intention to ensure that health promotion is appropriately and adequately resourced, the new scheme is also intended to allow the addressing of other locally agreed priorities, flowing either from central strategic intentions or from the identification of particular local needs. Many practices had already been undertaking worthwhile activity outside the scope of the core programme, and further developments should be encouraged when circumstances and resources permit.

In the first nine months of the new scheme's operation, from 1 July 1993 to 31 March 1994, transitional payments will be available to those practices offering a band three health promotion programme, which were earning more money under the previous health promotion clinic arrangements than they can now earn from band three activities and asthma and diabetes care programmes, so long as they are carrying out an approved transitional programme.

In the second year of the scheme, from 1 April 1994 to 31 March 1995, it is intended that money will be redeployed from the transitional fund, to fund new activity within the care programmes and to resource new and existing activity within locally agreed priorities, and by the third year of the scheme, the entire transitional fund will have been redeployed in that way.

Meanwhile, in the second year of the scheme, transitional payments will continue to be paid to practices which had been receiving them from the start of the new system, but at approximately half the rate paid in the first nine months.

Organization of programmes

Practices will have to apply for approval of their programmes on an annual basis, by 31 January each year, on form FP/HPP/1, and to report progress in their annual reports by 30 June. They also have to include mid-year summaries of their progress to date on form FP/HPP/2, with their applications for reapproval.

It is open to single-handed doctors and two doctor practices to collaborate with others to organize and offer a joint programme if they wish.

The information in the Red Book about health promotion and chronic disease management has been supplemented by extensive guidance for regional authorities, FHSAs, LMCs and practices, sent out by the Department of Health on 12 January 1993 (FHSL(93)3). The guidance emphasizes that the information required by FHSAs in order to determine whether the programme meets the Red Book criteria should not be excessive or repetitive. Many practices will have referred in their applications to protocols or guidelines already approved under the old clinic arrangements, or to readily available national clinical guidance.

FHSAs are required to consult LMCs on the way in which the guidance from the Department of Health is followed through locally. Such consultation is required on issues arising from *The Health of the Nation* and regional, DHA and FHSA strategies for meeting Health of the Nation targets which should be taken into account in developing health promotion programmes; on local factors relevant to the development of health promotion programmes, including the selection of priority groups; on the level of coverage to be expected, and whether variations from national guidance are justified by local circumstances; and on the shared care arrangements for chronic disease management. FHSAs may also consult LMCs on the approach to be adopted in relation to borderline or unusual cases (*see* Box 6.1).

Box 6.1: Consultation with the LMC

- Development of health promotion programmes in relation to *Health of the Nation* and strategic policy documents.
- Local factors relevant to programmes.
- Selection of priority groups.
- Level of coverage.
- Shared care arrangements for chronic disease management.
- Approach to borderline or unusual cases.

The Department of Health is taking an active role centrally and through the regions, in order to promote the fair and consistent application of the new arrangements throughout the country, and is encouraging dialogue at regional level between NHS management and the profession about the framework, its implementation and any inconsistencies in interpretation.

Annual reports and information requirements

The move from health promotion clinics to health promotion programmes is founded on a more population-based approach to preventive care. Some basic information on the practice population is needed to underpin these programmes, and is to be summarized in annual reports. Many practices already hold such information, but for some it will be a new task; practices without computers face a particular challenge.

The contents of annual reports have therefore been rationalized; some previous requirements have been pruned, including information about premises, staffing and referrals, so as to eliminate duplication of data available elsewhere. The aim is to concentrate on information needed to support the new programmes, building on basic information supplied by all GPs on the health of their practice population.

Additional information will be expected from GPs offering health promotion or chronic disease management programmes, including a commentary indicating whether progress on coverage levels has been as expected, whether changes in the programme have been or will be required, what audit has been carried out, and whether joint working with other individuals or agencies has occurred.

The degree of detail in which practices compile information will be influenced by whether or not they are computerized, their computer's reporting capacity, and their own needs and interests. Rates of progress towards comprehensive information gathering will vary, and in the first year of the scheme it is acceptable for practices starting from a low base to demonstrate good progress, if they cannot meet the information requirements in full.

The detailed information requirements are defined in the Red Book, while the Departmental guidance suggests methods of presenting the data. In summary, information will be collected on a head count basis—the numbers of patients given advice, offered interventions etc—rather than an activity basis—the number of clinic sessions—and will be broken down by age and sex.

7 Target Payments

Cervical cytology

GPs are no longer paid item of service fees for cervical cytology tests; instead payment is based on a system of target payments reflecting levels of uptake.

Eligibility

A GP will receive a target payment at the higher rate if, on the first day of each quarter, at least 80% of the eligible women on his or her list, aged between 25 and 64 (21 and 60 in Scotland), have had an adequate smear (taken by any source) during a period of 5.5 years preceding the claim. Women aged 25 to 64 are defined as those born between the second day of the same quarter 65 years earlier and the first day of the quarter 40 years later. For example, on 1 October 1993, the target population of women includes those born between 2 October 1928 and 1 October 1968.

A GP will be paid a target payment at the lower rate if at least 50% of the eligible women on the partnership list have had an adequate test.

When the scheme was initially proposed, target payments were to be calculated on an individual basis for each doctor, relating solely to the women registered on his or her list. However, the scheme was subsequently modified so that target payments were calculated on a partnership basis.

The actual payment depends on the number of eligible patients, compared with those on the list of the average GP, and the number of adequate smears taken as part of general medical services as opposed to those done in DHA or private clinics.

Who is excluded from the target calculation?

Women who have had hysterectomies involving the complete removal of the cervix are excluded from the total number of women on the list when calculating coverage. GPs should notify their FHSA of the number of women in the age group who have had hysterectomies, and the number of those women who have had an adequate smear in the preceding 5.5 years, and should inform it of any new cases. No other categories of women are excluded from the calculation.

Maximum sum payable

The maximum sum payable to a GP depends on the number of eligible women aged between 25 and 64 on the partnership list, compared with the average number of such women. The average number is calculated by multiplying 430 (the number of eligible women on the average GP's list) by the number of partners. The maximum sum payable is therefore:

$$\frac{\text{number of eligible women on partnership list}}{430 \times \text{number of partners}} \times \begin{array}{c} \text{maximum sum payable} \\ \text{to the average GP} \end{array}$$

Calculating the payment

The GP is eligible for the whole of the relevant payment if at least 80%, or 50%, of the eligible women have had adequate smear tests carried out by GPs as part of general medical services.

The smear test may have been undertaken by other doctors in the partnership or other GPs, for example if the woman was registered with another practice before joining the current GP's list. As long as the tests were adequate and carried out as part of general medical services, they are included. However, tests taken by a GP as part of work for which payment by a health authority or another source is received are excluded.

If any smears are repeated during the 5.5 year period, an adequate smear taken by a GP will take precedence over one taken by any other source for the purpose of calculating payments.

If the target is reached but the number of adequate smear tests carried out by GPs as part of general medical services is below the target number, the maximum payment is scaled down. The GP is paid that proportion of the maximum which the number of adequate tests holds to the target number.

Examples

The following two examples illustrate the target calculation and payment system.

Example 1: four-partner practice

Target calculation

Total number of eligible women aged 25–64
(hysterectomies excluded)   = 1440

Total number of women who have had an adequate smear
in the preceding 5.5 years   = 1200

$$\frac{1200}{1440} = 83.3\%$$

Higher target payment is achieved. The number of smears required to reach
the higher target (the target number) is 1152 (80% of 1440).

Calculation of maximum sum payable

$$\text{Maximum sum payable} = \frac{1440 \text{ (number of eligible women on partnership list)}}{430 \text{ (number of eligible women on average list)} \times 4 \text{ (number of partners)}} \times \text{Maximum sum payable for the average practitioner (80\% level)}$$

Calculation of payment

Total number of adequate smears = 1200
of which 800 done by GP or partner
         160 done by another GP
         200 done by DHA
          40 done privately.

Therefore 960 were undertaken under general medical services.

Maximum sum payable $\times \dfrac{960}{1152}$ = actual payment to each partner

Example 2: three-partner practice

Target calculation

Total number of eligible women aged 25–64
(hysterectomies excluded)   = 600

Total number of women who have had an adequate smear
in the preceding 5.5 years   = 330

$$\frac{330}{600} = 55\%$$

Lower target payment is achieved. The number of smears required to reach the lower target (the target number) is 300 (50% of 600).

Calculation of maximum sum payable

$$\text{Maximum sum payable} = \frac{600}{430 \times 3} \times \begin{array}{c} \text{maximum sum payable for} \\ \text{the average practitioner} \\ \text{(50\% level)} \end{array}$$

Calculation of payment

Total number of adequate smears = 330
of which 240 done by GP or partner
        45 done by another GP
        30 done by DHA
        15 done privately.

Therefore 285 were undertaken under general medical services.

$$\text{Maximum sum payable} \times \frac{285}{300} = \text{actual payment to each partner}$$

By April 1994 all FHSAs should have sufficient data on their computer systems to calculate entitlement to payments. Meanwhile, FHSAs may apportion tests of unclear origin in proportion to the known proportion of tests carried out by a GP for women on his or her list. For example, if the source of 12 tests is unclear and a GP has been responsible for taking the tests of 150 women on his or her eligible list of 192, then $\frac{150}{180} \times 12$, ie 10, of the unclear source tests will be allowed for payment.

An FHSA will also accept until 1994 information based on a GP's own records; GPs should use form FP/TCC to claim if the evidence from practice records indicates that a target has been reached. The validity of the claim may be checked by the FHSA.

Immunization for children aged two and under

A target payment system has replaced the previous individual payments for each immunization provided to children under the age of two.

Eligibility

A GP is eligible for a higher rate target payment if, on the first day of a quarter, the number of courses completed in each of the following groups of immunizations amounts on average to 90% of the number needed to achieve full immunization of all children aged two on his or her list. For the purpose of calculation, children aged two are defined as those born between the second day of the same quarter three years earlier and the first day of the corresponding quarter one year later, inclusive. For example, on 1 October 1993, the target population of children includes those born between 2 October 1990 and 1 October 1991.

Group one	Group two	Group three
Diphtheria ⎫ Tetanus ⎬ 3 doses Poliomyelitis ⎭	Pertussis 3 doses	Measles 1 dose OR Measles ⎫ Mumps ⎬ 3 doses Rubella ⎭

A GP will be eligible for a lower rate target payment if the average of courses completed amounts to 70% of the number needed for full immunization.

When the scheme was first proposed, payment was to be based on an individual GP's list; the scheme was subsequently modified so that target payments were calculated on a partnership basis.

Maximum sum payable

The maximum sum payable depends on the number of children aged two on the partnership list, compared with the average number.

The average number is calculated by multiplying 22 (the number of children aged two on the average GP's list) by the number of partners. The maximum sum payable is therefore:

$$\frac{\text{number of children aged two on partnership list}}{22 \times \text{number of partners}} \quad \times \quad \begin{array}{c}\text{maximum sum}\\\text{payable to}\\\text{average GP}\end{array}$$

Calculating the payment

The proportion of the payment due to the GP depends on the number of courses of immunization completed by doctors as part of general medical services as opposed to those completed elsewhere, for example at health authority clinics.

A course completed by other GPs (inside or outside the partnership) as part of general medical services will count towards the payment of the doctor making the claim. This means that, if a child who has had all the completing doses moves and registers with another practice, the new practice can count that child towards its target payment even though it provided none of the immunizations.

A course will be considered as being completed by a GP as part of general medical services if he or she gives the final immunization needed to complete cover for the diseases in that group. Thus in group one the completing immunization will be the third poliomyelitis, if the child has also had three doses of diphtheria and tetanus vaccine.

Method of calculation

The first step is to decide how many completing immunizations are needed to reach a target. Twenty children have 60 immunization groups; so 42 completing immunizations would be required to reach the 70% target, and 54 for the 90% target. If the calculation results in a fraction, the target will be rounded to the nearest integer (0.5 being rounded down).

Secondly, it is necessary to decide whether a target has been reached by adding the numbers of completing immunizations carried out in each of the three groups. Thus, completing immunizations in excess of the target number in one group can top up the number in another group.

Thirdly, if a target has been achieved, it is necessary to calculate the maximum sum payable, comparing the actual number of eligible children with the average number.

Fourthly, it is necessary to count the number of completing immunizations carried out by GPs as part of general medical services for the three immunization groups, so that the appropriate proportion of the maximum sum payable can be calculated. Only one completing immunization per child can be counted for each group. Where the number of completing immunizations in each group done by GPs as part of general medical services is greater than the number of children needed to reach the target level, the latter figure is counted. For example, if a partnership has 40 children aged two on its list, 32 have completed their immunizations in each of the three groups, and all the completing doses were given by GPs, then the 70% target has been reached. As the 70% target number is 28 children who have had completing immunizations, only 28 count towards the work done by GPs in each group. Therefore, the number of completing immunizations done by GPs is regarded as 28 + 28 + 28 = 84 (= 100% of the number needed to reach the 70% target).

Finally, the actual amount payable is then calculated by multiplying the maximum sum payable by the number of completing immunizations done as part of general medical services for the three groups added together, counted in the manner described in the previous paragraph, and dividing by the number necessary to achieve the appropriate percentage cover. As there are three groups, the number necessary to achieve the target is the appropriate percentage of three times the number of children concerned.

If a GP works for another body such as a health authority, any immunization carried out as part of this other contract will not count towards payment. Work done by employed or attached staff at the direction of a GP as part of general medical services is, however, counted for payment.

How to claim

Claims should be made on form PT / TC1 no later than four months after the date to which the claim relates. GPs should report details of all immunizations to the appropriate health authorities and also inform the FHSA of any health authority appointments they hold which involve immunization work.

Example: six-partner practice

On the first day of the quarter a partnership of 6 doctors has 120 children aged two on its list. All 120 have had complete courses of immunizations against diphtheria, tetanus and poliomyelitis. Sixty of the completing immunizations were given by the GP's own practice, 30 by another GP practice and 30 by a DHA clinic.

Ninety of the children have had complete courses of immunization against pertussis. Of these 48 were given by the GP's own practice, none by another GP practice and 42 by a DHA clinic.

Seventy-two of the children have been immunized against measles, mumps and rubella. Of these courses, 30 were given by the GP's own practice, 12 by another GP practice and 30 by a DHA clinic.

Step one: How many completing immunizations are needed to reach a target?

One-hundred-and-twenty children have a maximum of 360 completing immunizations.
The 70% target requires 252 completing immunizations.
The 90% target requires 324 completing immunizations.

Step two: Has a target been reached?

Group 1 (DT and P)	120
Group 2 (Pertussis)	90
Group 3 (MMR)	72
Total	282

The 70% target has been reached.

Step three: What is the maximum sum payable?

$$\frac{120}{22 \times 6} \quad \times \quad \begin{array}{c}\text{maximum sum payable to}\\ \text{GP with an average list}\end{array} \quad = \quad \text{maximum sum payable}$$

Step four: What proportion of the work needed to reach the target was done by GPs as part of general medical services?

Group 1	GP's own practice	60
	Another GP	30
	Total	90

but since 70% = 84 immunizations, this is treated as 84

Group 2	GP's own practice	48
	Another GP	0
	Total	48
Group 3	GP's own practice	30
	Another GP	12
	Total	42

Group 1	84
Group 2	48
Group 3	42
Total of completing doses regarded as carried out by GPs	174

Step five: How much is the payment?

Number of completing immunizations regarded as given by GPs = 174

Number of completing immunizations needed to reach 70% = 252

Payment per partner $= \dfrac{174}{252} \times$ maximum sum payable for 70% target

Pre-school boosters for children aged five and under

Just as target payments are available for immunization of children aged two and under, they are also paid for pre-school boosters for children aged five and under.

Eligibility

A GP is eligible for a target payment at the higher rate if, on the first day of each quarter, 90% of the children on the partnership list who are aged five have had reinforcing doses of diphtheria, tetanus and polio immunizations. Children aged five are defined as those born between the second day of the same quarter six years earlier and the first day of the quarter a year later. For example, on 1 October 1993, the target population of children includes those born between 2 October 1987 and 1 October 1988.

If 70% of the children under five have reinforcing doses then a target payment at the lower rate will be made. The payment to be made will depend on the number of eligible patients, compared with the average number, and on the number of boosters given by GPs as opposed to those given by others. A child will only be considered as fully immunized if he or she has received booster doses of all three vaccines. One or two vaccines will not count.

Maximum sum payable

The number of children aged five on the partnership list compared to an average list will determine the maximum sum payable. The average number is calculated by multiplying 22 (the number of children aged five on the average GP's list) by the number of partners. The maximum sum payable is therefore:

$$\frac{\text{number of children aged five on the partnership list}}{22 \times \text{number of partners}} \times \frac{\text{maximum sum payable}}{\text{to average GP}}$$

Calculating the payment

The amount payable depends on the level of cover achieved and the number of complete booster doses of immunizations given by GPs as part of general medical services. Those provided by other sources, for example health authority clinics, do not count. Boosters given by other GPs under general medical services—for example if a child is given the necessary boosters by a GP in one practice and then moves to another part of the country and registers with a new doctor—will be counted in the target calculation of the claiming GP. The child will be counted towards the new GP's target levels and not those of the doctor who gave the boosters.

The first step in working out the payment to be made is to decide whether 90% or 70% of the total number of children have received booster doses for all three vaccines. In calculating the 90% or 70% target number, fractions will be rounded to the nearest integer (0.5 being rounded down). If a child does not have all three boosters at the same time, no account will be taken of them until all three boosters have been given. The booster will count as having been given by whoever gave the third booster dose.

Secondly, if a target is reached, the number of booster doses given as part of general medical services is counted so that the appropriate proportion of the maximum sum payable can be calculated.

Thirdly, the actual amount is calculated by multiplying the maximum sum payable by the number of booster doses given under general medical services, and dividing by the number of boosters necessary to achieve the appropriate percentage cover.

Work does not count as having been performed by a GP as part of general medical services if he or she immunizes children under a paid contract outside the GMS system. Work done by employed staff or attached staff under the direction of a GP as part of general medical services will, however, be counted.

How to claim

Claims should be made to the FHSA on form FP/TPB no later than four months after the date on which eligibility is assessed.

GPs are responsible for reporting all immunizations to the appropriate health authority as soon as they are given. This allows health authorities to provide GPs with information to help them in claiming payments.

GPs are also responsible for reporting to the FHSA any appointment that they hold with a health authority which includes providing pre-school boosters.

8 Part-time Work in GP and Community Hospitals

Defining a GP or community hospital

A GP or community hospital is one without resident medical staff, where the first point of contact for medical treatment and advice (either routine or emergency) is a local general practitioner.

Methods of payment

There are three methods of payment as follows.

Clinical assistant sessions

The term 'clinical assistant' is not to be found anywhere in the terms and conditions of service for hospital medical and dental staff; however, the grade is covered by rules of appointment specified in paragraph 94 of the Terms and Conditions of Service of Hospital Medical and Dental Staff. A GP in the grade is responsible to a named consultant and, whilst working as a clinical assistant during a routine session, his or her overriding commitment is to the hospital service, not general practice. Thus, if a GP undertakes clinical assistant work, other arrangements have to be made to attend practice emergencies.

The clinical assistant grade is covered by NHS General Whitley Council regulations, and manpower approval is not required to establish a post of fewer than six sessions. Clinical assistant posts are normally offered on a 12-month fixed-term contract basis, and renewed annually. Emergency and on call duties should be specified in the contract, something which is almost invariably neglected.

Hospital practitioner sessions (*see* DHSS circular HC(79)16—August 1970)

Appointment to this grade requires four years' full registration with the General Medical Council and is subject to manpower approval. The post has to be advertised and applicants must be principals in general practice. A post at this grade cannot exceed the maximum of five sessions per week and the qualifications and experience of the post-holder will depend on the post itself and the views of the local consultants concerned. Like the clinical assistant, a hospital practitioner does *not* carry independent clinical responsibility; he or she is responsible to a named consultant. Terms and conditions of service are those of hospital doctors.

Staff fund arrangements (*see* DHSS circular HC(PC)(79)5—August 1979)

1 *Staff or 'bed' funds*. The 'bed fund' is a pool into which all bed fund and casualty earnings are paid. The distribution of this fund is agreed among the participating doctors and payments from the fund are superannuable. Only principals on the local FHSA list are appointed to the staff of a GP hospital with a bed fund. Doctors paid under the bed fund scheme are free to organize the paid work they do under the auspices of the fund. As independent clinicians, they are accountable to their peers on the medical staff committee. Bed fund payments are calculated according to bed occupancy, rather than the amount of time spent on the work.
2 *Casualty payments*. These are paid into the bed fund and are part of it. The clinical assistant pay rate is used to calculate the payments, but they are not connected to the clinical assistant grade. There are two components of the payments: a retention fee and an additional payment which reflects the number of attendances.
    The current retention fee (April 1993) is:

Monday to Friday, 12 hours per day	£1760 per annum
seven-day 12-hour service	£2465 per annum
seven-day 24-hour service	£4935 per annum

The payment related to numbers of new casualty attendances is based upon the clinical assistant pay scale, but this may be subject to local variation.

The arrangements for casualty payments do not require the attending GP to see all patients when they first attend; however, each patient should be seen by the doctor at some stage during the clinical episode. These arrangements enable a nurse to deal with minor problems, seeking advice and assistance from the GP as and when required. However, the GP must be prepared to attend *immediately* if requested to do so.

Contractual matters

The contract should specify who leads the team at the hospital. If a consultant is in overall charge, it should indicate how often he or she is expected to visit. If the hospital is consultant-led, the GP's post should be paid at either the clinical assistant or hospital practitioner grade. If there is a choice, the hospital practitioner grade may be more advantageous because it offers security of tenure and a higher level of pay.

The bed classification policy of the regional health authority should be clearly defined. There are many local variations with regard to the classification of GP and community hospitals.

The contract should also specify the duties and hours of work for clinical assistant and hospital practitioner posts. It is comparatively simple to calculate sessional payments for routine work, but far harder to calculate payment for out-of-hours work.

The hours during which casualty work is covered must be clearly defined. Some GPs, whose surgery is on the site of a GP hospital, find that during the hours nine to five they are not paid for casualty work, because the health authorities regard such work as part of general medical services. This interpretation is incorrect: casualty work of this kind is *not* part of general medical services.

Box 8.1: Contract checklist

The contract for sessional work in a GP or community hospital should include:

- the name of the employing authority
- the date employment commences and dates of any previous employment with which it is continuous
- a job description
- hours of work
- superannuation
- remuneration
- annual leave
- study leave
- maternity leave
- sick leave
- a definition of clinical responsibility
- substitution and deputizing arrangements
- medical indemnity
- period of notice of termination
- disciplinary procedure
- grievance procedure
- reference to the terms and conditions of service for hospital medical and dental staff, as appropriate.

A cautionary note of advice

GPs are advised to exercise great care before taking any steps to initiate changes to the contractual arrangements of their hospital posts. This cautionary approach is particularly apposite in the current climate of the NHS. Many GPs working in hospitals do not enjoy great security of tenure, particularly if they work for one or two sessions per week. The response of local management to a GP's proposals to change contractual arrangements may not be favourable; indeed, services may be reduced in response to a demand for increased remuneration. GPs should be aware that some NHS Trusts offer local contracts which do not correspond to nationally negotiated agreements, and which may not contain the same safeguards (eg annual pay increases).

Before raising any proposal with local hospital management, a GP should seek professional advice and assistance; otherwise he may unwittingly prejudice his long-term position. BMA members can obtain this expert advice and assistance from their regional offices. If working for an NHS Trust, a GP should also make contact with the Local Medical Committee (LMC) and Local Negotiating Committee (LNC), which will be in a position to negotiate with the Trust management on behalf of medical staff employed by it.

9 Other Income Sources

NHS general practice generates, in most cases, the majority of its income from the FHSA by means of fees, allowances and the various available refunds.

However, there is nothing to stop GPs, either personally or through their partnership, from earning additional income; indeed the vast majority of general practices do so to a greater or lesser degree.

The extent to which these other income sources apply to any given practice normally depends on such items as the nature of the locality and patients; the philosophy of the GPs and the commitment the partners are prepared to give to the practice. Nevertheless, such income is a useful and regular supplement for practices and frequently makes the difference between an averagely remunerated practice and one in which the partners are receiving incomes well above published levels.

Fees received by many practices include the following.

1 *Insurance reports and medicals*. Most practices receive a fairly regular source of income from reports and, in some cases, examinations on behalf of insurance companies which require information concerning the health of patients taking out life assurance policies. For expensive policies, a particularly rigorous examination may be required.
2 *Public service medicals*. Many practices receive regular payments for such items as attendance allowances or civil service medicals for certain patients. In some cases, GPs are appointed by a local public office to deal with such medicals and are paid separately from that source.
3 *Examinations and procedures on behalf of patients*. A steady but modest income can be earned from such items as HGV medicals for drivers, completion of BUPA referral forms, passport applications and numerous other items.

    Some GPs are uncertain about the fees they should charge for such work. Suggested fees are published on a regular basis both in medical journals and by the BMA. A notice should be placed in the reception area or waiting room so that patients can see the cost of such services.
4 *Cremation fees*. Many GPs receive income from signing cremation certificates and a fee is obtained for this. It is important that this is properly recorded and shown separately in the practice accounts. This is because the Inland Revenue can (and does) send representatives to

examine the books of undertakers and crematoria to obtain details of fees paid to GPs. The Inland Revenue is then able to cross-check with the GPs' accounts to see if these have been properly returned. Failure to do so has proved expensive for some practices and can lead, in extreme cases, to a full examination of the GPs' accounts, with potentially disastrous consequences.

5 *Police surgeon fees*. Some GPs are appointed police doctors, and are called to the scene of accidents to perform breathalyser tests, etc. For a practice that obtains such an appointment on a regular basis, the income received can be significant, although this is offset by the unsocial hours often required.

6 *Company medicals and retainers*. Some GPs obtain appointments with businesses. The work can be extensive, looking after the medical affairs of a large workforce. On the other hand, it may require only occasional attendance. In many cases, a retainer can be obtained which will give a regular source of income.

7 *Sundry cash fees*. It is important that any cash fees received in the surgery, for sundry certificates, passports or sick notes, are properly recorded and paid to the bank at regular intervals. If retained personally by the GPs, they must be declared to the Inland Revenue (*see* Chapter 17).

8 *Private patients*. Many practices attract private patients. This depends primarily on the locality, and to some extent on the practice policy. Some practices discourage private patients for reasons of conscience.

   If private patients are accepted, they should be dealt with in a business-like manner; accounts should be rendered at regular intervals, normally monthly or in some cases quarterly, and procedures should be instituted to ensure that payment is received with minimum delay. For larger private practices, a more complete credit control system may be required.

9 *Hospital appointments*. Some practices obtain appointments at local hospitals, as clinical assistants, casualty officers or for attendances at clinics. These part-time hospital appointments are normally taxed and care must be taken to see that the fees are paid into the practice account if that is the policy of the partnership. Earnings from appointments at local hospitals may be taxed at source, which can cause a problem in partnerships (*see* Chapter 39).

Partnership earnings

The partnership deed should define what are and what are not partnership earnings. This will depend on the policy of the partnership, but it should nevertheless be clearly set out in the deed (*see* Chapter 22).

Well organized partnerships, operating with a high level of financial discipline, usually insist that all medical earnings of the partners, from whatever source, are paid into the partnership account for division between the partners in agreed ratios. Failure to do so can give rise to disputes between partners.

10 Claiming Direct Refunds

A range of expenses paid directly by GPs for their practices are reimbursed directly to them, wholly or in part, by the FHSA. It is important that the procedure for making a claim is understood, to ensure that full refunds are received. It is also necessary for such expenditure to be grossed up in the accounts so that expenses are maximized in the event of their being examined as part of the Review Body sampling process (*see* Chapter 3).

General practice is the only profession inside or outside the NHS, which has this extremely beneficial system of direct refunds, by which GPs are effectively 'cushioned' against rises in expenditure during times of high inflation and periods of low pay increases. High cost items, such as rates and trainees' salaries, may be repaid in full.

It is, however, surprising how many practices fail to benefit fully from this system, usually because of inadequate claiming procedures which have lost practices many thousands of pounds.

All practices should therefore set up an efficient system for claiming these refunds. Where possible, responsibility for this should be delegated to the practice manager or one of her staff, who will be responsible for ensuring that correct claims are submitted and that accurate refunds are obtained from the FHSA. The SFA is the definitive reference and should be consulted when doubt arises. Relevant paragraphs in the SFA follow.

Rents

Paragraph 51. Where a practice rents a surgery from a third party, ie a landlord, the rent paid is normally reimbursed in full. However, in some cases GPs do not use the whole of the leased building for NHS purposes; in such cases a restriction is applied, and only a proportion of the rent is reimbursable. Where this applies the district valuer visits the premises and assesses the proportion of rent qualifying for refund.

The district valuer may consider the rent paid to be above the market rental value of the property, in which case a lower notional rent figure may be substituted. GPs do not, therefore, have a 'carte blanche' facility to pay out, and be refunded, an unlimited amount in rent. The amount paid must always be relevant both to the level of accommodation provided and known rental values.

GPs who own their own surgeries receive either a notional or cost rent allowance. These are dealt with at some length in Chapters 27 and 28.

Rates

Paragraph 51.13(b). GPs can claim a full refund of all rates paid on behalf of their surgeries. This normally includes:

* uniform business rates
* water rates
* water (metered) charges (paragraph 51.13(c))
* drainage rates
* sewerage rates.

The latter two items only apply in some areas. In some urban areas, a charge may be made by the local authority for disposal of trade refuse. Where this occurs, a refund should be claimed from the FHSA (paragraph 51.13(d)).

Rates will not be reimbursed where the rental includes a charge for rates.

Some practices choose to make payments of business rates by monthly standing orders, normally by 10 such payments between May and February. Care must be taken to see that these instalments are recovered on a regular basis, which is normally quarterly.

In some areas, FHSAs have agreed to make payments of this nature, normally business and water rates, direct to the local authority or water company concerned, without any cash passing through the practice. This is attractive to practices who consequently do not have to concern themselves with making payments or dealing with the claiming and receipt of the refund. However, it does impose on the practice an obligation to ensure that these figures are included on both sides of the accounts (*see* Chapter 18). The mere fact that they are not passed physically through the accounts does not mean that they can be ignored.

Ancillary staff refunds

Until 1990 it was common for practices to be refunded 70% of the gross salaries of all ancillary staff and 100% of the employer's share of the National Insurance contribution. However, this is no longer the case as payments are now subject to negotiation with the FHSA.

For the practice to qualify for a refund, ancillary staff may be engaged to carry out certain duties:

* nursing and treatment
* secretarial and clerical work, including records and filing

- receiving patients
- making appointments
- dispensing.

It should be noted that this scheme does not include salaries of cleaners, which do not qualify for a refund. Salaries of practice managers are generally held to fall within the qualifying parameters and, since April 1990, salaries paid to GPs' spouses normally qualify for a refund (*see* Chapter 43). Moreover, staff engaged in a wider range of duties—including physiotherapists, dietitians, counsellors, link workers, translators, etc—may also now qualify.

The system has changed significantly over recent years, as FHSAs must now impose cash limits on refunds of this nature. Practices should try to negotiate with the FHSA beforehand to ensure that their ancillary staff refund is maximized.

Where such cash limits are imposed, however, some FHSAs quote a standard figure for the ensuing year, which is paid in monthly instalments, regardless of the number of staff engaged by that particular practice. Different considerations do, however, apply in various parts of the country and practices should be aware of the policy of their FHSA.

GPs in health centres

Paragraph 53. There is no direct charge for rent and rates to doctors practising from publicly owned health centres (normally owned and administered by a district health authority).

Instead the payments are usually dealt with internally, without passing through the practice bank account. In such cases, it is important that the figure for rent or rates be obtained and included as an item of both expense and refund on both sides of the annual practice accounts. This serves the purpose of maximizing expenses in case the accounts are required for examination by the Review Body (*see* Chapter 3).

Similarly, some practices in health centres do not employ their own staff; they are administered and paid by the health authority. In such cases the doctor is normally charged a net percentage of staff salaries, with a full remission of National Insurance contributions. Again, it is necessary for this expenditure to be grossed up, in the case of salaries with 100% shown on the expenditure side and the appropriate percentage as a refund. National Insurance contributions should also be shown fully on both sides of the accounts. This information should be automatically supplied to the practice at regular intervals.

GP trainees

GPs who undertake the training of young doctors are paid a fee in the form of a trainee supervision grant.

For practice purposes, the GP trainee, during his year with the practice, is paid a salary based upon a scale negotiated from time to time and advised to the practice by the FHSA. This salary is paid to the trainee as if he were a normal employee of the practice, with the full range of PAYE and Class 1 National Insurance deductions being imposed.

A refund is, however, made to the practice of the amount of the gross salary, plus the car allowance, medical defence body subscription and the employer's share of the National Insurance contributions.

Training practices are dealt with in more detail in Chapter 32.

Car parking

In some urban areas, where it is necessary for the doctors to use a municipal car park, a refund of car parking charges can be claimed from the FHSA under a local agreement. This is normally in the form of a refund of fees charged for contract parking tickets.

Drug refunds

Many practices make claims for repayment of the costs of drugs dispensed or provided for patients. GPs should ensure that they make their claims on a regular basis. Refunds are normally made in arrears, often by as much as three months. Dispensing practices are dealt with in more detail in Chapter 33.

Computer grants

Paragraph 58. A scheme was introduced in 1990 whereby GPs can obtain a refund of part of the cost of installing computers in their practice, as well as for leasing and maintenance costs. This is dealt with fully in Chapter 20.

Payments on account

GPs can obtain by right monthly payments on account of all items described in this chapter, except rates, (unless paid by monthly standing order) or rent, which are normally repaid on presentation of the necessary receipt. It is particularly important in respect of ancillary staff and trainee refunds, that payment on account is received monthly, with a balance at the end of the quarter. If properly done, this could have a significant effect on the practice's cash flow position.

In all cases, care should be taken to ensure that refunds are claimed in an efficient and systematic manner, to ensure a prompt flow of cash through the practice. The responsibility for claiming refunds lies entirely with the practice, and it is not unusual to find practices failing to claim some or all of the items described, with significant effects on the earning levels of the partners.

A well drawn up set of practice accounts should show that refunds have been obtained, and the payment on one side should match the refund obtained on the other (*see* Chapter 16).

Abatement of direct refunds

The SFA in paragraphs 51.16 and 52.19, authorizes FHSAs to make a deduction or abatement from direct refunds in certain cases where it can be shown that fees from non-NHS sources amount to more than 10% of the gross practice income. Where two surgeries are in use, this percentage increases to 15%. Gross practice income is not clearly defined, but it is generally considered to represent the total income of the practice from all sources, including refunds, but excluding income from NHS sources other than that received via the FHSA, such as earnings from hospital appointments. The illustration of gross practice income, in the specimen accounts on pages 98–112, is from an example practice with a total income from all sources of £582 492. Any possible abatement of refunds would, for that example, be calculated as follows.

	Total income (£)	Non-NHS income (£)
Gross income, per accounts	582 492	
Income from appointments (Note 11)		61 466
Non-NHS fees (Note 12)		12 478
		73 944
Less: Interest, etc.	(1246)	
NHS appointments (Note 11): £9648 + £2645	(12 293)	(12 293)
	568 953	61 651

The proportion of non-NHS income using this formula is 10.8%, so the practice may suffer abatement of direct refunds. It should be noted, however, that this rule only applies to the use of wholly or partially financed NHS premises or staff for private purposes. The proceeds from non-NHS work carried out, for example, at the GP's home, can be omitted from the calculation.

In the case of the practice illustrated in Chapter 18, from which the above calculation derives (Note 11; page 105), a high proportion of the non-NHS income comes from work as a Police Surgeon. Therefore, provided the practice can convince the FHSA that NHS financed premises or staff are not used for this purpose, it should not suffer abatement.

11 Management and Efficiency in General Practice

IT has frequently been said—and will bear repeating—that efficient financial management is the key to the realization of acceptable levels of income in the general practice. Not only will this affect the partners who, as the key professionals involved, display their knowledge and skills in earning such an income, but also the other members of the primary health care team, whose support and effort are equally essential.

It has also been said that efficiency is an attitude of mind and that the practice which really wants to be efficient will succeed in its endeavour.

General practice is as much a business as the work of professionals outside the health care field, such as that of solicitors, accountants or architects who sell their professional skills with a view to profit. In the same way, the profitable business is likely to be the financially efficient one.

In general medical practice, this can readily be seen by comparing apparently identical practices between which there can nevertheless be a large disparity in levels of income.

Discrepancies in income levels in general practice are by no means unusual. On the one hand, one may find a highly efficient dispensing or training practice, with several outside appointments, some private patient earnings, maximum staff levels and the partners earning incomes in excess of £60 000 per annum. Even allowing for inflation, the number of 'wealthy' practices is likely to increase. Indeed, the introduction of the 1990 GP contract with its emphasis on capitation- and performance-based payments, has resulted in many more efficient practices earning levels of income previously unforeseen.

Such a practice is likely to be a highly efficient medium-sized business, with the partners all taking a share of executive responsibility, and the practice manager dealing with the day to day running of the practice, leaving the doctors largely to concentrate on their clinical duties to the ultimate benefit of patients.

At the other end of the scale, there may be an apparently identical practice, but where the partners take little interest in administration and operate on a shoe-string, with two or three part-time receptionists, no recognizable practice manager and little attention being made to the regular submission of item of service claims; the lack of attention is all too evident.

Those who are privileged to see the accounts of various doctors' practices from around the country will testify to the huge differences in incomes which can occur. Invariably, the difference between two apparently identical practices in financial terms is due to the quality of the management and the manner in which income is generated.

What then do we mean by financial efficiency and how can this be obtained? In medical practice, it generally falls into several categories:

1 the maximization of income levels, generally through item of service fees and target payments (Chapters 4 and 7)
2 the timely and accurate claiming of refunds (Chapter 10)
3 adequate staffing levels (Chapter 15)
4 control over expenditure levels, with proper budgeting procedures (Chapter 12)
5 a well maintained book-keeping system (Chapter 16)
6 computerization (Chapter 20).

Each of these are discussed in some detail in the chapters indicated.

Whilst it cannot be guaranteed that meeting these criteria will have an automatic effect on profits, the practice which gets all these right, and has the necessary will to maintain them at a high standard, has a far greater chance of attaining reasonably high income levels than one which does not.

The role of the practice manager

It is no exaggeration to say that a qualified, experienced and committed practice manager is probably the most important person in the efficiently run practice. She (or increasingly he) should be the equivalent of a company secretary, with control over the finances, administration, management and staffing of the practice below partner level. She should attend and participate in practice meetings and generally act as guide, philosopher and friend to her doctors.

The emphasis in the job title is on the word 'manager': the practice 'manager' should be the head of the team. Yet, in some practices the practice manager is not taken into the confidence of the doctors, and is thus excluded from the ultimate management function. She is treated as little more than a superior receptionist/secretary and has little part to play in the decision-making processes. This is ultimately to the detriment of the practice.

One of the more important tasks of the practice manager is the control of the practice finances; to ensure that these are run in an efficient and systematic manner, to maximize the practice income, keep a control on expenditure and hence increase the profitability of the practice.

Good management involves successful delegation of responsibility and the manager in general practice must be prepared, where necessary, to ensure that part of her workload is delegated to more junior staff, whom it will be more cost-effective to employ for that purpose.

Many practices fall into the trap of not adequately defining the practice manager's role; she may lack a full job description—or even, in some cases, a contract of employment—and may find herself taking conflicting instructions from different partners. She will therefore feel unappreciated and unfulfilled.

At the other end of the scale, a few enlightened practices have sought to give practical recognition of the importance of the practice manager's role by elevating her to partner status. Such a step, whilst generally to be welcomed, can create problems with regard to her taxation position, of liability in professional negligence cases, and in relations with other senior staff.

Training

The far-sighted practice will ensure that a comprehensive and progressive programme of training is in force, not only for the partners and practice manager, but for all members of staff: receptionists, nurses, secretarial and support staff. Regular courses are organized by Radcliffe Medical Press, as well as by AHCPA and AMSPAR, which can result in a recognized professional qualification.

12 Control of Expenditure

THE means by which practices can maximize their income, explored in Chapters 4–7, represent only one side of the equation in the quest for a financially efficient practice. Profit represents income less expenses and, whilst many practices are highly efficient in organizing their income and maintaining it at a high level, expenditure can easily get out of control. Many practices are subject to spiralling costs, which they make little effort to contain, and which inevitably have an effect on ultimate profit and hence the earnings of the partners.

The following example shows how one practice largely solved this problem.

	Year to 30 June 1992	Year to 30 June 1993
Gross income	405 791	430 138
Expenditure	198 946	192 468
Profit for year	206 845	237 670

This particular practice, through a drastic pruning of expenses, managed to increase its profit by 15%. However, this was at a time of low pay increases and without any guarantee that, unless rigidly controlled, costs can be maintained at a similarly low level.

Gross income rose by 6%, from £405 791 to £430 138. This is modest but acceptable, bearing in mind the financial climate in which it was realized. It is, however, in the field of expenditure saving that the practice has made an effort which has resulted in total costs falling by 3%. Profits for the practice (with five parity partners) have risen by over £6000 per partner over the year.

How did they achieve this? First, income was maintained at a reasonable level and this was an efficient practice that already had high earnings. The practice introduced strict budgeting procedures to control costs; the practice manager ran an efficient cash flow forecasting system; wages were pruned as far as possible, down to the level at which the cash limited refund came into force.

However, the most dramatic saving was in the cutting of relief service and locum fees. In the previous year, the practice had taken on a new partner but had not utilized this additional facility to save on fees of this nature. The doctors brought into force a revised rota system which ensured that not only were night visit fees maximized, but payments to locums and relief services were largely dispensed with. The cash flow forecasting system ensured that drawings could be taken when funds were available and this greatly reduced bank interest charges. Other significant savings were from accountancy fees, telephone and stationery costs.

Such a dramatic result is not possible for every practice, but the means by which it was brought about are not difficult to install. Given the necessary will, any practice can introduce economies of this nature.

Budgeting procedures

In a conventional business, which may be operated from several separate centres, the introduction of wide-ranging budgets is often a complex and time consuming procedure. In a typical general practice, however, such problems should not arise; keeping a control on outgoings is not unduly difficult, given the impetus and the co-operation of both the practice manager and the partners. Such a budget may be drawn up shortly before the start of each financial year, or as soon as the books have been balanced for any given year of account. It is suggested that this be done by the practice manager and agreed by the partners at the time. Budgeting should be an item on the agenda for a management meeting held at or about that time. For convenience, the budget may be drawn up for a period that coincides with the practice's accounting year. In any case, it should be approved and in force at latest by the end of the month following the last accounting year end. If, therefore, the practice accounts end in June 1993, a budget for the ensuing year should be in force by the end of July 1993.

Table 12.1 sets out a typical expenditure budget for a practice with a year end of 30 June. It shows the total budget for 1993/94, together with the actual and cumulative costs for the first two months of the year, ie July and August 1993, illustrating how it is possible to make a running check of expenses by this means.

It is important that not only is the budget drawn up at the proper time, but it is controlled and regularly monitored throughout the year covered. There is no point whatever in having a budget if this is then filed away and forgotten about.

There will always be unforeseen items which cannot reasonably be taken into account at the time the budget is prepared, and some practices choose to include a contingency fund to cater for such items. There may be unforeseen repairs required to the building; a partner may be required to take sickness or maternity leave which involves the partnership in additional

Table 12.1   Extract from an expenditure budget control sheet: year to 30 June 1994

	Annual budget (£)	July 1993 Actual (£)	August 1993 Actual (£)	To date (£)
Drugs and appliances	2000	–	100	100
Locum fees	3000	–	–	–
Deputizing	1000	50	50	100
Equipment hire	1500	200	150	350
NHS levies	500	–	–	–
Training costs	600	50	30	80
Books and journals	100	–	20	20
Staff salaries (inc. NIC)	30 000	2500	2350	4850
Trainees' salaries	15 000	1250	1250	2500
Staff welfare	1000	100	50	150
Recruitment costs	500	–	80	80
Rates and water	5300	400	400	800
Light and heat	1500	–	150	150
Repairs and renewals	2000	500	100	600
Insurance premiums	800	–	200	200
Cleaning and laundry	2000	200	200	400
Garden maintenance	500	50	20	70
Printing, stationery and postage	1800	500	200	700
Telephone	4800	500	200	700
Accountancy	4200	–	–	–
Bank charges	200	–	100	100
Legal charges	200	–	100	100
Sundry expenses	1500	200	100	300
TOTAL BUDGETED COSTS	80 000	6500	5850	12 350

locum expenses; there may be exceptional increases in telephone, cleaning and heating charges. Where such a contingency is operated, however, it should be treated as precisely that and the facility not abused.

It is essential to maintain control that the budget is reviewed at regular— no more than monthly—intervals, and the partners should be made aware of any exceptional variants.

It should go without saying that such a budget cannot be efficiently formulated or monitored without an efficient and up to date book-keeping system, which is considered in more detail in Chapter 16.

13 Cash Flow: Problems and Principles

MOST businesses are able to maintain an acceptable and regular cash flow through the systematic issue of invoices and statements, together with an efficient system of credit control.

Few of the problems generally associated with this system affect the typical practice, where most income is received on a regular basis, with monthly and quarterly remittances from the FHSA. It is with regard to outgoings from the practice account and, in particular, drawings by individual partners, that control of cash flow is most important.

The cash flow forecast

Whilst a historical record of cash passing through the practice is by no means a bad thing, the systematic production of cash flow forecasts for up to a year hence is even more useful. These should look at the manner in which income will be received and outgoings paid, by which it will be possible to control the balance on hand at any given date.

It should be emphasized that such a forecast is not a projection of profit, but merely of the movements of cash, which for this purpose includes the practice bank accounts. Opinions vary as to exactly how long a period such a forecast should cover, but it is usually taken that it will cover each accounting year; thus if a practice makes up its accounts to 30 June annually, then during May or June 1993 it should be considering the preparation of a cash flow forecast for the year to 30 June 1994.

This is not necessarily as difficult as it sounds, particularly for a practice which has had an established system over many years and whose book-keeping system is such that the required information can be produced with a minimum of delay. It is, of course, essential that such a forecast is reviewed on a regular basis. This should be done at least quarterly, but preferably monthly. Many practices now present cash flow forecasts on spreadsheets included in computer programs. Where this is done, amendments can be made easily, avoiding the need for complex mathematical calculations.

A practice may make a good profit and the financial accounts may apparently show a healthy financial position, yet it may still have cash flow problems. This will probably be due to the slow receipt of items of income or excessive drawings by the partners. This will only come to light through the completion of a cash flow forecast, which not only shows how much cash is received, but when it is received and when paid out.

Once prepared, such a forecast may be used for the planning of major expenditure or as a basis for a presentation to lending institutions in support of applications for loans or mortgages. It also facilitates the preparation of partners' drawings, enabling these to be dealt with in a far more logical and realistic manner than might otherwise be possible. The control of balances held on the bank account can prevent unnecessary overdrafts, and hence result in a significant saving in bank interest charges.

Drawings

Systems of drawings are many and varied, and are outlined in more detail in Chapter 26. It is essential that a proper system of drawings be implemented and this is an integral part of a cash flow forecast. Some practices prefer to equalize payments to partners, primarily for their own convenience and ease of personal budgeting, whereas others will pay out on the basis of funds accumulated in the bank account at the end of each month or quarter.

Whichever of these, or other, systems is used, a properly managed system of cash flow forecasting offers the partners a clear idea of how much they are likely to be able to draw month by month or quarter by quarter.

Figure 13.1 shows a typical practice's cash flow forecast for April to March, and predicts the opening and closing bank balances for each month. This particular forecast envisages large withdrawals by the partners during June, at the same time that substantial amounts are paid out in respect of rates which are not reimbursed until the following month. On this basis, a decision could be made to spread partners' drawings more evenly over the year, in an attempt to eliminate the need for a substantial overdraft from June to November.

Receipts	April	May	June	July	Aug	Sept	Oct	Nov	Dec	Jan	Feb	March	Total
NHS fees/allowances	9500	9500	11 365	9800	9800	13 652	9800	9800	12 653	10 000	10 000	13 652	129 522
Ancillary staff refunds	438	1294	1066	1003	1070	1107	856	908	927	927	998	1080	11 674
Trainee refunds	640	640	640	720	720	720	720	845	845	845	845	845	9025
Rent and rates	750	750	750	2975	750	750	750	750	750	750	750	750	11 225
Drugs refunds	–	–	–	192	–	–	70	190	1296	–	16	–	1764
Insurance exams	300	78	250	220	443	401	249	419	426	777	215	312	4090
Cremation fees	21	–	21	–	23	42	–	–	42	21	–	–	170
Appointments	208	208	208	208	208	208	208	208	208	208	208	208	2496
Sundry fees	62	42	163	–	–	315	27	63	–	412	–	–	1084
Total receipts	11 919	12 512	14 463	15 118	13 014	17 195	12 680	13 183	17 147	13 940	13 032	16 847	171 050

Figure 13.1 A sample cash flow forecast: (i) receipts

Payments	April	May	June	July	Aug	Sept	Oct	Nov	Dec	Jan	Feb	March	Total
Staff salaries & NIC	617	1822	1502	1412	1507	1559	1206	1279	1305	1305	1406	1521	16 441
Trainees salaries	640	640	640	720	720	720	720	845	845	845	845	845	9025
Locum fees	432	512	245	–	315	645	315	545	215	150	450	215	4039
Relief service fees	70	35	–	70	75	40	62	52	120	–	–	75	599
Drugs & instruments	172	–	–	56	200	1300	–	20	–	–	42	23	1813
Rent and rates	750	750	3725	750	750	750	750	750	750	750	750	750	11 975
Repairs and renewals	72	–	84	12	160	–	–	51	20	–	–	61	460
Petty cash	100	100	100	100	100	100	100	100	100	200	100	100	1300
Loan interest	423	389	532	423	398	452	396	401	463	363	431	462	5133
Loan repayments	500	500	500	500	500	500	500	500	500	500	500	500	6000
Accountancy fees	–	1500	262	–	500	352	300	–	123	–	–	273	3310
Insurance	–	–	–	–	–	750	–	–	–	840	–	–	1590
Lighting and heating	–	98	–	55	46	–	–	62	59	–	–	–	320
Bank chgs & interest	–	–	96	–	–	162	–	–	73	–	–	106	437
Telephone	–	–	839	–	–	433	–	–	926	–	–	519	2717
Drawings	7500	7500	12 636	7900	7900	7900	7900	7900	7900	7900	7900	7900	98 736
Sundries	72	–	735	42	78	24	924	–	–	2460	260	107	4702
Total payments	11 348	13 846	21 896	12 040	13 249	15 687	13 173	12 505	13 399	15 313	12 684	13 457	168 597
Net cash flow	571	–1334	–7433	3078	–235	1508	–493	678	3748	–1373	348	3390	2453
Opening bank balance	1604	2175	841	–6592	–3514	–3749	–2242	–2734	–2056	1691	318	666	1604
Closing bank balance	2175	841	–6592	–3514	–3749	–2242	–2734	–2056	1691	318	666	4056	4057

Figure 13.1 *contd.* A sample cash flow forecast: (ii) payments

14 Business Planning for the General Practice

THE concept of business planning for general practices has come to the fore in recent years, to some degree encouraged by two factors:

1 the extension of the DTI Enterprise Initiative Scheme to general practice in late 1990
2 the introduction of GP fundholding; those practices proposing to enter the scheme have been required to prepare a business (or practice) plan looking at the manner in which they propose to go about it.

Business planning has, in this manner, only recently been extended to general practice, and many GPs have been reluctant to take it on, chiefly because:

1 they do not wish to trust their private affairs to outside consultants
2 they believe that consultants cannot possibly know as much about their business as they do
3 they resent the likely cost.

In fact, none of these concerns have proved justified in most cases.

What is a business plan?

By and large, a business plan represents a forward-looking, systematic approach to running a business, with which many GPs agree in theory but are reluctant to implement in practice. Only by looking ahead, and setting down in clear and concise terms the path it expects to follow in the next few years, can any business run in an entirely successful manner, whether it be a giant multinational corporation, a corner shop or general practice.

Such a plan may lead to either a consolidation or a decision to change course. Reduced to its essentials, a business plan should set out to answer the following questions:

1 Where are we now?
2 Where do we propose to be in five years' time?
3 How are we going to achieve this?

In practice, a period of five years is normally considered applicable to plans of this nature, although this could be varied by agreement.

The plan should incorporate a number of features outlined in this book: cash flow forecasts (Chapter 13); expenditure budgets (Chapter 12); maximization of income (Chapters 4–7); examination of performance by statistics (Chapter 19); staffing levels (Chapter 15), and several others.

With the introduction of business values into general practice, the process of business planning is becoming more widespread, although many practices still hesitate in going down this road. However, the advent of GP fundholding, and the recruitment of more professionally able and qualified business managers to run practices, make it likely that business planning will gather force in future years.

Who should do the work?

Many practices resist the idea of introducing outside consultants, preferring to save the cost and do the work themselves. One must question whether this is a misguided policy; an outside consultant can offer a degree of detachment not always possible if the plan is prepared in-house; internal political factors can be kept at bay and, indeed, an independent mediator may at times be able to resolve them.

The consultant should be prepared to sit down, both separately and collectively, with all the partners, and look at their ambitions and aspirations, the type of medicine they wish to practice and the level of earnings they wish to enjoy, etc.

He or she should be both experienced and knowledgeable about the affairs of general practice, understand how GP finances work and, above all, be used to dealing with non-corporate businesses, particularly partnerships.

What will it cost?

There are two main types of plan prepared for the general practice, and it is important to understand how each of these might be financed.

1. The DTI Enterprise Initiative Scheme

This scheme has been in force for many years, but has only been available to GPs since 1990. The basis of the scheme is that a business consultant is engaged by the practice, normally from a list of specialists registered with the

DTI, to prepare the plan; fees are fixed by negotiation between the practice and the DTI so that they cannot subsequently be increased. A practice is therefore fully aware of its commitment before the work commences.

Such an assignment normally lasts 5–15 days, charged at a daily rate. Experience tends to show that a full and satisfactory plan cannot be prepared in less than 15 days.

The cost to the practice need not necessarily be large; normally one third of the cost is paid by the DTI. This subsidy is extended to half the cost in certain development areas, which change from time to time but currently include all the inner London boroughs and parts of South Wales, Scotland and North East England.

Figure 14.1 shows the likely net cost of a DTI business plan, covering a 15-day assignment for a six-doctor practice in a development area. After deduction of the 50% DTI grant and tax relief, the average cost per annum per partner is about £80—a bargain when one considers the benefits that such a plan might introduce.

	£
Fee: 15 days @ £450 per day[1]	6750
Add: VAT @ 17.5%	1182
	7932
Less: 50% payable by DTI	3966
	3966
Less: Tax relief @ 40%[2]	1586
	2380
Average net cost per partner	397
Average cost per partner per annum[3]	79

[1]Costs can vary in different areas.
[2]The level of tax relief is variable.
[3]Assumes currency period of five years.

Figure 14.1   Example costing of a DTI business plan for a six-doctor practice in a development area (15-day assignment)

2. The fundholding management allowance

Business plans for fundholding practices are discussed in Chapter 34.

It should, however, be noted that the residual cost to the practice of a DTI business plan cannot be met out of the fund-holding management allowance. It is a condition of the DTI Enterprise Initiative Scheme that the net cost falls on the business under review, and is not met from another source of public funding.

What should it contain?

The exact structure and contents of the plan are a matter for initial discussion between the consultant preparing the plan and the partners for whom it is intended. In the case of DTI plans for a large busy practice, it is virtually impossible to look at every aspect of the practice's function within the prescribed period of 15 days. It is therefore necessary to be selective and to highlight problems which are apparent; indeed, those which may have caused the partners to consider going through the planning process in the first place.

All plans should, however, contain:

- a mission statement
- a SWOT analysis
- an action plan
- profit projections and cash flow forecasts
- current activity levels and targeting of achievements
- environmental issues, including the standard of the practice premises, administration, organization and staffing matters.

Above all, the plan should contain precise guidance as to exactly how it will be implemented.

The mission statement

This briefly sets out the overall philosophy of the practice and the partners, as well as taking into account the wishes of the staff and patients. For example, a mission statement for a typical practice could read:

'. . . to provide a high level of patient care, taking into account the practice's commitment to the National Health Service, whilst at the same time maintaining an acceptable level of income for the partners and staff.

We believe this can best be implemented within the context of a friendly and informal practice, in which patients have regular access to the doctor of their choice, and that offers a range of quality services and maintains a high quality practice team.'

The SWOT analysis

An essential part of the plan is the discussion and establishment of the 'strengths', 'weaknesses', 'opportunities' and 'threats' applied to the practice. This involves exploring how strengths and opportunities could be benefited

Strengths

- good premises
- high quality of young partners
- loyal and committed staff
- high level of activity in health promotion clinics
- large list sizes generate good capitation income
- commitment to the NHS
- practice fully computerized

Weaknesses

- difficulty in meeting targets
- low level of proceeds from night visits
- high expenditure on deputizing
- branch surgery generating insufficient income
- senior partners of similar age
- difficulty in patient communication due to lower social class
- some partners not interested in expanding practice
- long waiting times annoy patients

Opportunities

- new housing estate being built
- additional marketing activity
- apply for additional partner
- formulate new rota to do more night visits
- utilize available space more efficiently
- introduce staff training scheme

Threats

- three senior partners likely to retire within next five years
- practice manager likely to move away within two years
- patients leaving through difficulty in obtaining appointments,
- effect of national policy on GPs' income levels

Figure 14.2   A typical SWOT analysis

from, and how weaknesses and threats could be counteracted. Figure 14.2 shows a typical SWOT analysis for a sizeable practice.

Implementation and monitoring

The completed plan should set out the current situation and look at how proposed aims can be achieved over a five-year period. As a long term plan, it should be flexible enough to incorporate changes that will inevitably be necessary in response to environmental or political factors.

It goes without saying that the plan should not be left to gather dust in a drawer, but should be monitored on a regular basis; the proposals, which should have been accepted by the partners before the plan is finally formulated, should be implemented on the dates projected.

How to go about it?

Those GPs who feel they would benefit from the business planning process (and there cannot be many who would not) should initially consider using the DTI business planning initiative under the Enterprise Initiative Scheme. If this fails, or cannot be introduced for some reason, they should approach their FSHA to see if help is available from that direction. Finally, they are strongly advised to appoint a consultant specializing in this field, who would initially meet the partners, draw up a plan of action and terms of reference, and set out details of likely costs.

It should then be possible for the practice to go ahead with the business plan to the benefit of all concerned.

However, it should be noted that the present DTI scheme is due to end on 31 March 1994, and there is no guarantee that it will be renewed.

15 Employing Staff

A GP's staff are probably his most important asset. He is highly dependent on them; they are the first point of contact for patients; they run the administrative systems and carry out a wide range of clerical, executive and clinical tasks. The GP, as the employer, is liable for their acts and/or omissions. However, as a doctor, the GP is more vulnerable than other employers, being subject to 'disciplinary' procedures specific to medicine and general practice (including the FHSA's Medical Service Committee and the GMC's disciplinary procedures). Disciplinary procedures can be triggered by an act or an omission by a GP's employee.

In addition, the costs of employing practice staff comprise a sizeable proportion of a GP's total expenditure. Although hitherto 70% of spending on salaries has been reimbursed, the introduction of cash limits on FHSA spending, together with the increased discretion FHSAs are allowed to exercise when determining where and how much to reimburse GPs directly for their staff, will eventually lead to considerable variations in the pattern and level of direct reimbursement among individual GPs and practices, and also among FHSAs.

The neglect of staff matters by GPs is evident in the recruitment, selection and training of staff; these are often undertaken on an *ad-hoc* basis. Although efforts have been made to inform GPs about the need to provide written contracts of employment for their staff, many practice staff do not have written contracts and many of the contracts that have been issued are either incomplete or substantially incorrect. Generally, many GPs are unaware of the legal responsibilities and obligations they carry as employers. Ignorance is no defence if a legal dispute should occur and the GP has to defend his or her actions in an industrial tribunal or court of law.

Why is there such widespread neglect of employment matters? GPs have been trained primarily as clinicians and have acquired little, if any, formal training in the skills and knowledge required to run a small business. Indeed, many GPs regard the managerial and administrative side of general practice as an intrusion upon their time, interrupting the primary task of providing clinical services to patients.

This neglect of employment matters is common among small employers, who do not have the time and resources to ensure that their legal responsibilities and obligations are properly fulfilled. One apparent reason for this neglect is that, because staff matters are essentially concerned with human relationships, it is inappropriate to allow the formality of the law to intrude. This excuse is frequently deployed to explain such failures as ignoring the legal rights of a pregnant employee, lacking any health and safety arrangements at the surgery premises, and failing to provide written contracts of employment.

GPs, who would never contemplate entering into a commercial contract without satifactory legal documentation (eg the purchase of a car, the acquisition of a bank loan or the negotiation of a lease for their premises), become party to an employment contract that is vague and undocumented, even though this contract may involve a financial commitment of a comparable size and may lead to substantial damages if mistakes occur in its application.

Within the confines of a single chapter it is possible only to highlight some key issues arising from the employment of practice staff. More detailed reading is recommended on all these topics, and in particular every GP should have a copy of *Employing staff* by Norman Ellis, published by the British Medical Journal. This book provides a comprehensive and readable account of all the issues with which a GP needs to be familiar.

Any BMA member is strongly urged to contact the BMA regional office if he requires advice or assistance, particularly if he anticipates a problem. Often, GPs consult the BMA when it is too late to resolve what would otherwise have been avoidable. For example, a dismissal may have been initiated by a practice and an incorrect (and often illegal) procedure or reason for the dismissal is pursued. If help is sought too late, the BMA's staff can assist only in damage limitation.

Recruitment and selection of staff

A GP should adopt a more formal approach to recruiting and selecting staff than is generally found in small businesses. Good recruitment and selection procedures improve the running of the practice, by reducing staff turnover for example. If the appropriate people are chosen, they are likely to give good and loyal service; inappropriate personnel will leave voluntarily when they find more suitable employment, leave involuntarily if dismissed, or more often remain in the practice providing an indifferent or unsatisfactory standard of service. The following key points on the recruitment and selection of staff should be noted.

1 When the vacancy occurs, write a job description, prepare a profile of the person required and advertise for applicants.

2 Interview a shortlist of suitable applicants, keep notes of impressions of candidates, and do not inadvertently enter into verbal contractual commitments during the interview.
3 Inform all applicants of the outcome; the letter offering the job should state the date on which employment begins and cover the main headings of the contract.
4 Ensure that on appointment the employee has a clear understanding of her duties.

The practice manager should participate in the recruitment process; she will have to train and work with the new member of staff.

Training and induction of staff

Although it may seem self-evident that any new employee should be properly trained and introduced into the practice, it is surprising how often employers neglect or forget this essential task. Staff are a vital asset to any general practice and a GP should ensure that they are able to contribute to the best of their abilities. If adequate induction and training are not provided, a GP could be in an insecure position if disciplinary action ever has to be taken.

The induction of a new employee will depend on the practice's circumstances and the resources which can be devoted to it. Induction need not be elaborate, but it should be planned in advance and undertaken with care. The practice manager and other supervisory staff should be involved, although only one person should have overall responsibility for induction. The completion of induction does not mean that training has ended. GPs should encourage their staff to attend training and continuing education courses.

The 1990 contract specifically requires GPs to ensure that their health professional staff (ie those who provide health care services to patients) are properly qualified and receive regular training.

The contract of employment

A contract of employment exists as soon as an employee shows her acceptance of an employer's terms and conditions of employment by starting work, and both employer and employee are bound by the terms offered and accepted. Often the initial agreement is verbal not written, but within two calendar months of an employee starting work the employer is legally obliged to provide a written statement detailing the main terms of employment with an additional note on disciplinary procedures. (This requirement does not cover staff who normally work fewer than eight hours a week.)

This statement must contain:

1 names of parties to the contract
2 the date employment began and a statement about continuity of employment
3 job title
4 pay
5 hours of work
6 holiday entitlement and holiday pay
7 sick pay
8 pension
9 notice of termination
10 grievance, disciplinary and appeals procedures.

It is sensible to prepare and issue a comprehensive contract of employment that covers all these subjects. (BMA members can obtain a model contract of employment from BMA regional offices.)

Attention paid to preparing a correct contract of employment ensures that unforeseen and unwanted disputes do not arise. The preparation and agreement of the contract should ensure that the employer is reasonably familiar with his legal responsibility and obligations and has not unknowingly acted contrary to these at the outset. Moreover, if any dispute should arise and a GP has to defend personnel practices and policies, the doctor's position is greatly strengthened if it can be shown that he acted in good faith and had taken reasonable steps to act in accordance with the law.

Finally, a written contract may have to be changed; no difficulties should arise if the correct procedure is adopted and the substantive reason for the change is 'reasonable'.

Dismissal

In general, employees who have not completed two years' continuous employment by the date on which dismissal takes place, or who work fewer than 16 hours a week unless they have been employed continuously for at least eight hours a week for more than five years, cannot complain of unfair dismissal. This also applies to employees who have reached the normal retirement age for their employment or, if there is none, men or women who have reached 60 years.

The risk of a successful claim of unfair dismissal (which can involve compensation payments of many thousands of pounds) can be largely avoided if the procedure adopted is both fair and reasonable, and the reasons for the dismissal are also fair and reasonable. An employer may have to justify his or her actions so it is wise to keep detailed documentation throughout. Finally, any BMA member contemplating a dismissal, but who is uncertain about how to approach it, should not hesitate to contact his BMA regional office for advice and assistance at the earliest possible opportunity.

Statutory maternity rights

Most practices employ only a small number of staff, and the majority of these are women. The employment rights of the expectant mother are intricate and stringent. Thus, any employer with a small number of staff may be faced with serious administrative problems if a member of staff becomes pregnant.

An expectant mother has hitherto acquired three distinct employment rights:

1 not to be unreasonably refused paid time off work for antenatal care—applicable to all employees irrespective of their length of service
2 to receive statutory maternity pay (SMP) if she has 26 weeks' recent continuous employment with an employer and normal weekly earnings above the NI lower limit
3 to return to work with her employer after a period of absence on account of pregnancy and confinement.

The third right is acquired by an employee only if she has been continuously employed for at least two years and normally works for 16 or more hours a week, or has been with the practice for at least five years if she normally works for 8–16 hours a week.

The Government introduced new employment legislation in 1993, which gives all women employees two new statutory maternity rights:

1 not to be dismissed for reasons connected with pregnancy or childbirth
2 14 weeks paid maternity leave (irrespective of length of service or number of hours worked per week).

This area of employment law is the most complex for employer and employee. It is vital that any GP should obtain detailed guidance on how to ensure that an employee obtains her statutory maternity rights. The Department of Social Security (DSS) has published a free booklet explaining SMP; every GP should obtain a copy of it. Any mistake, even if it is due to ignorance or a misunderstanding of the law, could lead to a tribunal case and a costly compensatory award. Industrial tribunals are assiduous in upholding the rights of pregnant employees and have imposed severe penalties in cases where unfair dismissals have occurred because of pregnancy; more rulings of this nature are likely when the new rights have been implemented.

Statutory sick pay

The statutory sick pay (SSP) scheme establishes a minimum entitlement for sick pay for most employees. Every employer is required to pay sickness benefit as the agent of the Government, but the decision on when sick pay should be paid lies primarily with the employer rather than the Department of Social Security (DSS).

The main features of SSP are as follows.

1 NI sickness benefit is no longer payable for most sickness absence; instead SSP is paid directly by the employer.
2 SSP is paid in the same way as normal pay and is liable to deductions for income tax and NI contributions.
3 Entitlement to sick pay does not depend on previous NI contributions or previous service with the employer.
4 Married women paying the reduced contribution and part-timers are entitled to SSP provided that their earnings are above a specified figure.
5 The total SSP that may be received from one employer for one or more periods of sickness cannot exceed 28 weeks' worth; after 28 weeks state benefit may be claimed from the DSS.
6 The employer has to decide whether sick pay is due.
7 The employer (depending on size) can deduct either all or 80% of the amount paid out in SSP from remittances to the Inland Revenue of NI contributions, although no deduction can be made for any amounts paid in error.
8 SSP is paid at two rates according to the average weekly earnings of the employee.

The rules of SSP are complicated (but fortunately not as difficult as those that apply to maternity rights) and need to be applied correctly. Every GP should have a free copy of the DSS's booklet *Employers' manual on statutory sick pay.*

Health and safety in the surgery

The Health and Safety at Work Act requires an employer, including a self-employed person, to provide and maintain a safe working environment, and it has established powers and penalties to enforce safety laws. The main thrust of the Act is to make both employers and employees more conscious of the need for safety in all aspects of the working environment. The most important duties are those that any employer must fulfil to staff, ie all that is reasonably practicable to ensure their well-being. The words 'reasonably practicable' are important; what is expected of an employer depends on the size of the business and the resources available. Thus, in general practice, a larger partnership carries a heavier burden of responsibility than one that has fewer staff and resources.

The law requires an employer to provide information, training and supervision for staff on health and safety matters. Unless there are less than five staff, the employer must provide a written statement of general policy on health and safety and the arrangements for implementing this. It can be included in the written contract of employment.

The GP also has a duty to ensure the safety of anyone who enters the surgery or health centre, including patients, visitors, building contractors, tradesmen and health authority staff. If the premises are owned by a private landlord or the DHA, the licence or lease may impose this duty upon these other parties and they may also be liable if there is an accident.

16 Basic Book-keeping and Accounts

GENERAL practice is big business: even a small practice has a turnover running well into six figures. Most conventional business enterprises of this scale employ skilled accounting staff, so the problem of inadequate records would not apply. Doctors, however, are notoriously bad at keeping records.

Most doctors have had no financial training. On entering general practice, however, they could become, within a relatively short period, equity partners in a medium-sized business enterprise. GPs then have to participate in decisions affecting: the finances of themselves, their partners and their staff; employment and staffing; budgeting and controls; taxation, insurance, banking and investment.

Financial decisions, which have to be taken regularly in all medical practices, are virtually impossible without access to well-maintained and comprehensive accounting records. Such records should be kept, or supervised, by a competent practice manager and they should form the basis of the practice's financial reporting facility, as sensible business decisions cannot be made without them.

The prime reasons for having book-keeping records are:

1 to identify items of income and to highlight means by which this can be maximized
2 to monitor expenditure and, through successful budgeting, control costs and economize (Chapter 12)
3 to draw up meaningful cash flow forecasts (Chapter 13)
4 by means of the above, to maximize profits and hence the income of the partners
5 to comply with a clause in the partnership deed, which may specify that 'proper book-keeping records shall be kept'
6 if applying for fundholding status, to increase the likelihood of acceptance
7 to have records available in the event of enquiry by the Inland Revenue into the practice's affairs
8 to make a possible saving in accounting fees.

Sometimes outside accountants keep the books of a practice, but this is likely to be expensive. It is uneconomic to have a professional person dealing with routine book-keeping records, as GPs have the facility to recover a proportion of the costs of employing practice staff, including clerical staff such as book-keepers. An accountant's fees are not recoverable, either wholly or partly, from the FHSA, and they include a 17.5% VAT charge. However, most accountants will be happy to advise staff on methods of writing up the books, and if necessary teach them how to do so.

The types of book-keeping records that should be kept are discussed below.

The main cash book

The main cash book is the basis of the practice accounting system. Unlike the petty cash book, it records the receipts and payments of monies paid into and withdrawn from the practice bank account. This is *not*, therefore, the same thing as a ledger.

The vast majority of the transactions passing through the practice will go straight into the partnership bank account. Cheques will be received and banked and the majority of FHSA income may arrive by direct credit; cheques will be drawn at regular intervals for running expenses, staff wages, partners' drawings etc.

All of these should be recorded in the cash book, always up to date and maintained at regular intervals. Figure 16.1 shows a possible layout for an analysis cash book.

The member of staff responsible should aim to:

- balance the book periodically, at least monthly
- reconcile this balance regularly with the bank account statements.

Buying the book

There are a number of excellent analysis books on the market, eg the 'Guildhall' and 'Cathedral' systems and several other series offering a large variety of columns at each opening. Make sure you buy the right book; if in doubt, take along someone knowledgeable to advise you.

How many columns?

There should be sufficient columns of both receipts and payments to reflect adequately the transactions of the practice. This will, of course, vary according to the nature of the practice.

For instance, in a large practice with a significant income from dispensing work, private patients or outside appointments, the type and variety of

Figure 16.1 The GP's cash book: recommended column headings

Receipts

1993	Details	TOTAL	NHS	Appointments	Insurance Exams, etc	Sundry fees	Other receipts
Jan 1 Balance b/forward		2,653 94					2653 94
H.Smith – fee	5 –					5 –	
ABC Insurance Co	9 –				9 –		
DEF Insurance Co	9 –				9 –		
3 GHI Insurance Co	9 –				9 –		
JKL Insurance Co	9 50				9 50		
Income tax repaid	127 85						127 85
County College	350 –			350 –			
MNO Insurance Co	9 50				9 50		
5 Private certificate	2 –					2 –	
7 B.J.Funeral–Crem fee	16 50	547 35				16 50	
11 PQR Insurance Co	9 50				9 50		
STU Insurance Co	9 –				9 –		
13 Loamshire County Council	15 –					15 –	
14 Mr Jones – fee	20 –					20 –	
Mr Brown – fee	25 –					25 –	
Mr Williams – fee	30 –					30 –	
17 XYZ Nursing Home	500 –			500 –			
ABC Insurance Co	9 50				9 50		
18 DEF Insurance Co	9 –				9 –		
Mr White	20 –					20 –	
20 Loamshire FHSA Rent & Rates		2,350 –	2,350 –				
GHI Insurance Co	9 50				9 50		
Mrs Green	35 –					35 –	
22 Loamshire Hospital Clinical Assistant	108 96			108 96			
23 JKL Insurance Co	9 50	809 96			9 50		
24 Loamshire FHSA							
25 Trainee refund		3,647 94	3,647 94				
JKL Insurance Co	9 50				9 50		
ABC Insurance Co	9 50				9 50		
Mr Black	56 –					56 –	
Mr Blue	25 –					25 –	
28 Sundry cash takings	55 –	171 50				55 –	
cremation fee	16 50					16 50	
31 Loamshire FHSA Monthly advance	7,250 –	7,250 –	7,250 –				
Ancillary staff	1,300 –	1,300 –	1,300 –				
	£18,724 69	14,547 94	958 96	121 –	321 –	3781 79	

Payments

1993	Cheque No.	Sub No.	TOTAL	Salaries	Drugs & instruments	Trainee payments	Locum fees	Rent and rates	Lighting & Heating	Cleaning	Telephone	Petty Cash	Repairs & rentals	Partners drawings	Tax reserve transfers	Sundries
Jan 1 Dr Jones locum	635.46 S.O.	1	100 –				100 –									
Transfer			1,200												1,200 –	
2 Building Society	47	2	85 76													85 76
Fire Insurance	48	3	2,575 –													2,575 –
3 Accountancy fees	49	4														
PAYE/NIC Month 9			897 40	651 10		246 30										
4 Smart Drug Company	50	5	35 65		35 65											
Electricity Board	51	6	152 75						152 75							
Mrs Jones: cleaner	52		20 –							20 –						
Petty cash	53		50 –									50 –				
6 Water Board	54	7	65 35					65 35								
9 Surgery rent	55	8	1,750 –					1,750 –								
Gas Board	56	9	97 50						97 50							
11 Post Office: Telephone	57		267 45								267 45					
Mr Brown: Plumb repair	58		25 –										25 –			
ZYX Instrument Co	59		15 50		15 50											
15 Dr Jones locum	60		150 –				150 –									
22 Cleaning materials	61		27 50							27 50						
Coffee	62		10 75													10 75
24 Legal charges	63		250 –													250 –
25 Petty cash	64		50 –									50 –				
31 Mrs V Wiliams	65		268 45	268 45												
Mrs J Smith	66		139 54	139 54												
Mrs B Jones	67		235 46	235 46												
Mrs D Johnson	68		226 92	226 92												
Mrs S Green	69		137 50	137 50												
Mrs A Watson	70		197 45	197 45												
Mrs M Robinson	71		226 45	226 45												
Mrs L White	72		57 50							57 50						
Dr N Hunt: trainee	73		858 75			858 75										
Borough Council & rates	S.O.		357 50					357 50								
Staff pension scheme	S.O.		500 –													500 –
Dr Grace	S.O.		2,200 –											2,200 –		
Dr Hobbs	S.O.		2,000 –											2,000 –		
Dr Bradman	S.O.		1,950 –											1,950 –		
Dr Hutton	S.O.		675 –											675 –		
			17,856 13	2,082 87	51 15	1,105 05	250 –	2,172 85	250 25	105 –	267 45	100 –	25 –	6,825 –	1,200 –	3,421 51
Balance c/forward			868 56													
			£18,724 69													

income will be such that more columns will be required than in a more basic practice.

Where necessary, advice should be sought on column headings.

All entries should be entered in a total column, as well as one of several analysis columns. Suggested column headings each side (receipts and payments) are listed in Boxes 16.1 and 16.2.

Box 16.1: The GP's cash book: recommended column headings—receipts

1 *Details:* all individual items of amounts paid to the bank in a single banking, eg 20 cheques of £20 each.
2 *Totals:* eg £400 from details above, plus any direct credits by the FHSA or other bodies.
3 *NHS fees and refunds:* all monies received from the FHSA, eg monthly advances, quarterly cheques, rent, rates, ancillary staff and trainee repayments.
4 *Outside appointments:* from schools, hospitals, nursing homes etc, who pay regular fees to the practice. It may be helpful to keep a separate column for any fees taxed at source.
5 *Insurance examinations*
6 *Sundry fees:* any payments which do not fall under the other headings. (Where justified by volume, it may be desirable to have a separate column for fees from private patients.)
7 *Other:* eg tax repayments, transfers from other bank accounts, leave advances, improvement grants, funds introduced by the partners, etc.

Box 16.2: The GP's cash book: recommended column headings— payments

1 *Cheque no.*
2 *Receipt no.:* the serial number of the receipted account for this particular payment. These should be numbered consecutively in a file maintained for that purpose.
3 *Total:* all payments passed through your bank account, including those charged directly by the bank, eg bank charges and standing orders. Amounts entered into the total column should also go into one of several analysis columns (or into several columns where one cheque covers separate items).

Box 16.2: *continued.*

Analysis columns

4 *Staff salaries:* payments to ancillary staff, *not* to partners or other doctors, or cleaners. Also enter amounts paid in respect of PAYE and NI contributions each month.

5 *Drugs and instruments:* for dispensing practices, payments to drug suppliers; otherwise all sundry payments for these items.

6 *Trainee payments:* all net amounts, plus PAYE and NI contributions.

7 *Locum fees:* including relief service payments.

8 *Rent, rates and water:* all payments including those refunded by your FHSA.

9 *Lighting and heating*

10 *Cleaning:* payments to cleaners, their PAYE and NI contributions, and cleaning materials purchases.

11 *Telephone:* surgery bills and partners' personal accounts, if relevant.

12 *Repairs and renewals:* building repairs, plumbing and electrical work, repairs to equipment etc, but *not* improvements or extensions or purchases of new equipment.

13 *Partners' drawings:* either use one column for each partner or enter all partners' drawings in the same one (these are not salaries and should not be shown in the salaries column).

14 *Building society interest:* some practices operate a tax reserve system, by which transfers are made monthly to a building society account.

15 *Sundries:* normally items which occur with insufficient frequency to justify a separate column, eg accountancy fees, bank charges/interest, transfers to tax reserve accounts, purchase of new equipment, insurance premiums, etc.

Direct debits and credits

These comprise receipts that are paid directly into the practice bank account by a third party, and payments made by standing order or direct debit.

Direct credits may be advised to you by your FHSA or insurance company, and can be entered into the cash book at that time; otherwise they should be entered when they appear on your bank statement.

Where direct debits are known to be occurring monthly, an entry can be made in the cash book at the appropriate date; otherwise enter them when you receive a bank statement.

All such items must be entered in the total column and the appropriate analysis column in the cash book.

Balancing the cash book

First check the mathematical accuracy of the entries you have made. Add up the total column and the various analysis columns, for both receipts and payments. It can be helpful to do this in pencil until you are satisfied that the figures are correct. A 'cross cast' can then be made, ie check that the total of all the analyses columns equals the total of the 'total' column (*see* Figure 16.1).

Then compare the totals of the receipts and payments columns and strike a balance; this should reflect the effective balance in the bank on a particular date. However, although this is the true balance, it is unlikely that it will be identical to that shown on the bank statement: an explanation of why and how to reconcile the bank balance is given below.

Cash book summary

	£
Balance b/fwd at 1 October 1993	1763.40
Add: Receipts for month	29 930.55
	31 693.95
Less: Payments for month	13 410.04
Balance per cash book at 31 October 1993 c/fwd	18 283.91

Reconciling the bank

It is essential to check the cash book entries against the monthly bank statement, and to reconcile the balance shown.

The steps to achieving this are:

1 Obtain the relevant bank statement(s).
2 Check the credit entries on the bank statement, by comparing entries on the right-hand side with your receipts total in the cash book. Some entries in the cash book may not appear on the bank statement until the following month; these are called 'late credits'.
3 Check the payments (left-hand column) as above. Monies paid out, which do not appear on the current month's statement, are called 'unpresented cheques'.
4 Ascertain the balance shown in the cash book.

5 Rule off the bank statement entries on the same dates.
6 List the late credits.
7 List the unpresented cheques.
8 Write down the month-end balance on the bank statement, and add to this the 'late credit' items to make a sub-total.
9 Subtract the total of the unpresented cheques from the sub-total.

The figures should then reconcile. If they do not, a repeat check should be made to identify the cause of the difference.

If there is an overdrawn balance on the bank statement, the procedure should be reversed, by adding the unpresented cheques and deducting the late credits.

Bank reconciliation

		£	£
Balance per bank at 31 October 1993			5369.38
Add: Outstanding credits			15 000.00
			931.63
			462.50
			21 763.51
Less: Unpresented cheques	054668	262.50	
	054669	342.70	
	054670	191.00	
	054671	150.00	
	054672	981.30	
	054673	982.40	
	054674	569.70	
			3479.60
Balance per cash book at 31 October 1993			18 283.91

Box 16.3: Tips for writing up and balancing the cash book

- Always keep up to date: it is easier to enter three or four cheques per day than all the month's cheques at once.
- Add up each page as you finish it.
- Leave the top and bottom lines on each page vacant for the totals and brought forward figures.
- Be methodical: establish a routine that suits you and stick to it.
- Be consistent: always enter the regular items in the same column from month to month.

Box 16.3: *continued.*

- Rule off at the year-end (say December 31) and leave two or three pages for late entries.
- If your accountant takes the accounts away for two or three weeks at year-end, it may be advisable to use different books for alternate years; alternatively, use a loose-leaf cash book so that pages can be easily extracted.
- Enter on each cheque counterfoil the full details, eg 'Mr Brown: plumbing repairs: £5'.
- Zeros in the pence column confuse matters when adding up; use dashes instead.
- Always enter the date on the first entry of each day, and show the year at the top of the page.
- If, when checking against bank statements, items do not correspond, make inquiries with the bank immediately; if you delay, they may no longer have the information at hand.
- Do not attempt to reconcile the bank statement at longer periods than one month.
- When reconciling a bank statement, *always* start with the bank balance and then adjust as indicated above.

Salaries and wages

Full records of all calculations of staff salaries and wages must be kept. Where this is done 'in-house' entries are usually made in a ruled book showing:

- gross salary
- deductions for:
    PAYE
    Class 1 NIC
    pension contributions (if applicable)
- net salary
- SSP/SMP (if applicable)
- Class 1 NIC (employer's share).

The amount paid to the employee should correspond with the figure shown in the 'net salary' column.

Some practices calculate their salaries using a computer program which can be efficient and cheap. Several organizations now offer computerized payroll management for those practices without such facilities. Such companies can relieve the GP or practice manager of extra work and can make arrangements for direct bank transfers into the accounts of the employees concerned.

Computerized accounts

Some practices have chosen to adopt a book-keeping system based on a specialized computer program (see also Chapter 20). GPs embarking upon such systems should ensure that they suit the requirements of the particular practice and that they are designed to cater for the different demands of general practice.

Figure 16.2 shows suggested headings for a computerized cash book in a typical three-doctor practice.

DRS MORRIS, AUSTIN AND RILEY:
CASH BOOK COLUMN HEADINGS

Receipts

Main column heading	Sub-column

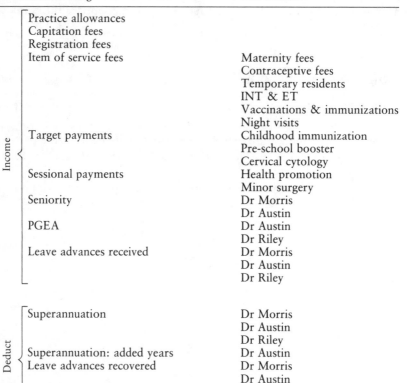

FHSA quarter statement

Income

Practice allowances
Capitation fees
Registration fees
Item of service fees | Maternity fees
| Contraceptive fees
| Temporary residents
| INT & ET
| Vaccinations & immunizations
| Night visits

Target payments | Childhood immunization
| Pre-school booster
| Cervical cytology

Sessional payments | Health promotion
| Minor surgery

Seniority | Dr Morris
| Dr Austin

PGEA | Dr Austin
| Dr Riley

Leave advances received | Dr Morris
| Dr Austin
| Dr Riley

Deduct

Superannuation | Dr Morris
| Dr Austin
| Dr Riley

Superannuation: added years | Dr Austin
Leave advances recovered | Dr Morris
| Dr Austin
| Dr Riley

NHS levies

Drugs refund
Rent & rates refunds
Ancillary staff refunds
Computer refunds
Hospital appointments
Other appointments
Insurance examinations
Cremations
Private patient fees
Sundry fees
Miscellaneous

Figure 16.2   Suggested cash book column headings: computerized accounts

Payments

Main column heading	Sub-column
Drugs and instruments	
Locum & relief service fees	
Hire and maintenance	
Practice replacements	
Medical subscriptions	
Medical books & journals	
Courses and conferences (Drs)	
Ancillary staff	Salaries
	PAYE/NIC
Staff expenses	Staff training expenses
	Recruitment costs
	Staff welfare
Rent & rates	
Insurance	
Lighting & heat	
Repairs & renewals	
Cleaning & laundry	
Postage & stationery	
Telephone	
Accountancy fees	
Bank charges & interest	
Capital expenditure	
Drawings	Dr Morris
	Dr Austin
	Dr Riley
Partners' tax	Dr Morris
	Dr Austin
	Dr Riley
Partners' NIC	Dr Morris
	Dr Austin
	Dr Riley
Loan repayments	
Petty cash	
Transfers to other a/c	
Sundries	

Figure 16.2: *continued*

17 Looking After the Petty Cash

ALL practices have cash passing through the surgery on a regular basis.

Firstly, one should consider what exactly is meant by petty cash. It literally means coins and bank notes, either received by the practice from patients as fee income or available in the form of a float, from which sundry cash disbursements can be made. These two aspects of petty cash in the average general practice should be kept entirely distinct.

The basic record for all cash transactions is the petty cash book, with the cash on hand on any given date being maintained in one or two petty cash boxes specifically used for that purpose.

The maintenance of an efficient and well regulated system of petty cash recording is an integral part of the practice's book-keeping arrangements. Whilst we may not be talking about large amounts of money, it does build up and, if it is not properly and efficiently recorded, can result in a great deal more trouble than it is worth.

Sundry cash receipts

It cannot be emphasized too strongly that any fees received in cash, whether for certificates, cremation or sundry, should be properly accounted for and paid into the practice bank account without deduction.

The incorrect notion persists that these fees are in some way 'perks of office' which need not be accounted for and which the doctor is entitled to put into his pocket without paying tax. Nothing could be further from the truth; such fees are the income from his profession and it is essential that they are fully accounted for, both for accountancy and taxation purposes.

Cremation fees, for instance, have been traced by the Inspector of Taxes and doctors have been asked to pay tax upon then, sometimes for several years in arrear. Such a liability, which may include interest and penalties as well as the tax loss, can amount to many times more than the tax 'saved' in the first place.

Cash receipts of this nature should always be collected and paid periodically into the practice bank, at the same time as routine payments of cheques to the bank. Many practices retain cash in a special tin for a week or a fortnight, or until they reach an agreed sum, eg £50.

Much depends on the circumstances of the practice and the volume of fees received, but a policy should be established and strictly adhered to.

The petty cash book

It is strongly recommended that a separate book (*see* Figure 17.1) be kept to record the sundry fees received, not only as a routine record but also to enable the practice manager to check whether particular fees have been received.

	Sundry Cash Receipts - May 1993	Fees		Other		
May 1	Mr Brown – fee	2	50			
	Mr Smith – examination	5	85			
	Mrs Green – private patient	7	50			
2	Mr Jones – certificate		50			
	Staff telephone – refund			3	75	
	Mrs Harrison – private patient	5	25			
	XYZ Insurance Co – examination	7	00			
4	Dr Williams – locum fee	10	00			
	£	38	60	3	75	
	Paid to Bank 5/5/1993 £	42	35			

Figure 17.1   A specimen page from a sundry cash receipts book

The book should have a separate column for recording receipts of a non-fee nature and it is suggested that a separate column also be maintained for recording cremation fees.

Cash should be collected in a cash tin retained for this purpose only, which is cleared fully when the periodic bankings are made, as outlined above.

The mixing of sundry cash receipts of this nature with cash retained for payment of sundry petty cash items should be strongly discouraged.

Cash payments

A separate cheque should be drawn periodically from the bank for sundry small payments, based upon an average weekly or monthly expenditure and replenished from time to time by a cashed cheque drawn on the practice bank account.

This too should be kept in a separate cash tin maintained for payment purposes. Doctors and staff requiring cash for any purpose should be asked to complete a petty cash voucher or submit a receipt.

Once made, all such payments should be regularly and systematically recorded in a petty cash book used only for this purpose. This should ideally be in the form of an analysis book, which should be regularly added up, balanced and reconciled with the cash held in the tin.

A specimen page from a typical payments petty cash book is shown in Figure 17.2.

Receipts, in the form of cash withdrawn from the bank, should be shown on the left-hand (or debit) side. Payments should be shown on the right-hand (or credit) side, being entered once in the payments (or 'total') column and again in the most appropriate analysis column.

The headings of the various analysis columns depend largely on the circumstances of the practice, but again they should be totalled periodically and, if the entries have been made correctly, the sum of the total of the various analysis columns should equal that of the payments column. These can all be totalled monthly and a balance carried forward to the start of the following month.

A test balance can be taken at any time, merely by finding the difference between the running totals of the receipts and payments columns. This should then be compared with the cash held in the tin and any difference investigated. Differences may well occur, usually for entirely innocent reasons; a payment might have been omitted from the petty cash book or an incorrect entry made.

RECEIPTS		PAYMENTS		Postage		Stationery		Partners National Insurance		Cleaning		Repairs		Locum Fees		Refreshments		Sundries	
32	97																		
		21	95	11	95			10	–										
		5	75			5	75												
		4	50							4	50								
40	–																		
		5	50							5	50								
		1	25															1	25
		6	80													6	80		
		10	–											10	–				
		4	75									4	75						
		23	60	10	–			13	60										
		2	65			2	65												
		5	25													5	25		
50	–																		
		1	50															1	50
		4	50															4	50
		6	50							6	50								
122	97	104	50																
				21	95	8	40	23	60	16	50	4	75	10	–	12	05	7	25
		18	47																
£ 122	97	122	97																

Figure 17.2   A few days' entries in a typical payments cash book

---

Box 17.1: Petty cash recording

Do:

- keep the cash proceeds from cash fees separate from cash used for making payments
- record cash fee income and pay into the practice bank account regularly
- make petty cash payments from a float withdrawn from the bank for that purpose
- record payments in an analysis cash book
- total the columns for each month and balance them
- reconcile the balance regularly with cash held in box
- ensure that petty cash drawn from the bank is recorded identically in both the petty cash receipts book and the main cash book (*see* Chapter 16).

Don't:

- mix up proceeds for cash fees with sundry cash payments
- keep inadequate records
- fail to count the cash regularly and check the balance.

Security

A few practices entirely eliminate the need to keep funds for payment of sundry cash items; it is certainly good policy to try and keep them at as low a level as possible. For instance: all staff wages/salaries should be paid either by bank giro credit or monthly cheque; postage stamps can be bought by cheque periodically from the post office; and classic petty cash items, such as milk deliveries, groceries and stationery, can all be converted to monthly accounts. If these are excluded, the need for substantial levels of cash in the surgery is very much reduced, enabling a far higher level of security and a reduced temptation to thieve.

18 Making Sense of Practice Accounts

VIRTUALLY all medical practices have a statement of accounts prepared on an annual basis so that the accounts are drawn up to a fixed accounting date each year. Most practices employ a specialist accountant to act for them in several different capacities. The duties the accountant should perform for the average medical practice are discussed in Chapter 49, but perhaps one of his main functions is the preparation of the annual accounts.

Some GPs question the need for accounts and feel that they are paying large amounts of money in professional fees for a document that they do not really need and which they may not fully understand. The purpose of this chapter is to examine the reasons why accounts should be drawn up and then to explain how they can be read and understood.

The major reasons why accounts are so necessary to the GP and his practice are listed in Box 18.1 and discussed in detail below.

1 *Tax*. Accounts are essential for agreeing the tax liability both of the partnership and the individual partners. This equally applies in the case of a sole practitioner.

   If accounts cannot be produced, the GP or his accountant will be unable to substantiate the level of profits upon which tax assessments are based, and he could find himself paying far more tax than necessary.

2 *Loan finance*. It is often necessary to produce a set of accounts when approaching banks or other lending institutions to borrow money. This is the case irrespective of whether the money is for a surgery development project or for the personal use of an individual partner, such as for the purchase of a private house or car.

3 *Practice management*. A well drawn-up set of accounts, giving valuable information concerning the profitability of the practice, is essential when determining the success of the practice in financial terms; as a base for formulating future budgets and calculating drawings; and when taking decisions on the admission of new partners.

4 *Income sources*. Accounts drawn up on this basis may highlight additional means by which the practice can generate income, from both NHS and non-NHS sources. This is important bearing in mind the manner in which GPs' projected income is calculated, with emphasis on efficiency and specified targets. It is therefore important to consider the level of income realized, as outlined in detail in Chapter 19.

5 *Cost economies.* A look at a logically drawn-up schedule of practice expenses for a year may help partners to identify means of cutting costs and hence increasing profits (*see* Chapter 12).

6 *Partnership deeds.* In a practice with a properly drawn-up partnership deed, there will be a clause requiring annual accounts to be drawn up, specifying the accounting year-end, that a professional firm of accountants will be used (and its name) and that the accounts must be signed by the partners as a true record (*see* Chapter 22).

7 *Capital and current accounts.* In many partnerships the allocation of these is complex (*see* Chapters 30 and 31) and it is essential that they be controlled in order to preserve fairness between the partners. Again, this is specified in many partnership deeds, but only by the production of regular and comprehensive annual accounts can control be effectively maintained.

8 *New partners.* Accounts can be an aid to recruiting suitable new partners, who may decline to join a practice which cannot produce a set of accounts from which they can ascertain their likely future earnings (*see* Chapter 25).

Box 18.1: Why do GPs need accounts?

- To agree practice tax liabilities.
- In support of applications for loan finance.
- As an essential management tool.
- To highlight possible new income sources.
- To make expenditure economies.
- Required by partnership deed.
- For equity between partners.
- To inform new partners.
- To make appropriate arrangements when a partner leaves.

Choice of year-end

Many practices have established year-ends and do not seek to change them. However, in some cases, particularly when new practices are being set up or a sole practitioner takes over from a retired doctor, there is an opportunity to decide a year-end for future use. It is suggested that several criteria be taken into consideration.

1 More accurate accounts, and hence more meaningful figures, tend to result from accounts prepared to a conventional quarter-end, ie 30 June,

30 September, 31 December and 31 March, because all NHS finances are organized on a quarterly basis. Where other year-ends are in force, it may be necessary to make apportionments and estimates which may not be entirely accurate.

2 For tax planning purposes, it is preferable to have accounts with the earliest possible year-end within the accounting year. For many conventional businesses, including those of dentists and private doctors, an April year-end is beneficial, but for GPs a June year-end is generally considered to be the most suitable.

3 Once a year-end is established, it may be changed if the taxpayer (and the partnership) wishes, but it is essential that knowledgeable professional advice is taken to ensure that there is no detriment in terms of tax payable.

How to read a set of accounts

Pages 98–112 show a typical set of parnership accounts for a six-doctor GP partnership. A statement of this type should ideally be prepared by the practice accountant each year, as soon as practicable after the accounting year-end. The accounts themselves are of a style frequently published and correspond to the style of publications issued by the Institute of Chartered Accountants. They also provide for all recommendations regarding the layout of accounts—chiefly concerning the 'grossing up' principle—in the Red Book.

Most accounts prepared for general practices, particularly large practices, are long and complex. Many GPs feel that their accounts are made unnecessarily complex. In fact, GPs' accounts are complex because the modern practice is complex, with its business activities spread over a number of separate functions. The partner should have greater cause for concern if his accounts did not fully reflect all the financial transactions of the practice over the year.

The accounts should be designed to take into account several aspects which are unique to general practice, and it is important that the following points are understood when reading the accounts.

1 *Comparative figures.* On pages 99 and 100, which set out the profit, income and expenditure of the practice, it will be seen that the column on the right-hand side gives comparatives with the previous year's figures. These should always be shown in a set of accounts so that trends in income and expenditure are apparent. This also applies to the balance sheet on page 101 and the various supporting notes on pages 103–10.

2 *Profit for the year.* Page 99 shows that the partnership has realized a total profit for the year of £348 633, an increase of 7.5% on the figure of £324 229 shown for the previous year. It is important that the concept of profit is understood; this is the means by which businesses finance themselves and, in the case of general practice, from which the partners earn their living.

3 *Income.* Page 100 sets out details of the income earned by the partnership during the year, through NHS fees, refunds and income from outside the NHS. Again, it is easy to obtain a comparison with the previous year.

4 *Payments.* Page 100 also shows the payments made by the practice during the year, and the manner in which the expenses have been divided, and further details are set out in the notes following.

5 *Profit-sharing.* Page 99 shows how the partners have been remunerated.

In this case (Note 3) there were two changes in the partnership during the year. On 30 September 1992, Dr Orange, who previously had a share of the profits of 16%, achieved partity at 20%. On 31 January 1993, Dr Black retired and on the following day a new partner, Dr Grey, was introduced to the practice, with a 12% share of profits. As this is by no means uncommon in GP partnerships, it is important that the profits for the year are allocated between these separate periods in such a way that no partner loses out through this process.

6 *Separate profit-sharing periods.* For many years it was accepted practice to allocate profits on the basis of income and expenditure recorded in each separate profit-sharing period in force during a single year of account. This was both time-consuming and expensive, but was considered to be essential if an accurate allocation of profit was to be achieved. To a large degree, the situation changed with the advent of the 1990 GP contract, by which the incidence of practice allowances (*see* Chapter 19) was greatly reduced. Thus the profits of a partnership became less dependent on the number of partners.

Practices have subsequently allocated profits on a time apportionment basis. This has avoided the additional cost of producing accounts on an actual basis, and appears to be acceptable to GPs. The accounts of the sample practice, to which I refer, have been prepared in this manner. The lower part of Note 3 shows that the total profits for the year available for allocation (£314 397) have been allocated on a monthly basis between the various profit-sharing periods in force. The profits shown in each of these individual periods have then been allocated between the partners' profit-sharing ratios as applicable to each separate period.

7 *The balance sheet.* This sets out, on page 101, the financial position as at any given date. It is normal practice for the accounts to be drawn up to

the same date each year, in this case 30 June 1993. The balance sheet gives details of the assets and liabilities of the practice and, importantly, the manner in which the capital has been provided by the partners.

Similarly, the investment of the partners in the fixed assets and the working capital of the practice is represented by their capital accounts (Note 21, page 109), and the overall figure of £80 000 calculated as set out in Chapter 31, page 189.

This concept of capital in medical partnerships is complex, but it is necessary to understand it fully in order to understand GPs' partnership accounts.

8   *Notes.* It is common for a number of items in the balance sheet and else-where to be set out in notes to the accounts—*see* page 103.

9   *Surgery ownership and income.* Note 16 (page 109) indicates that the practice owns its own surgery, which, in the balance sheet, is shown to be worth £631 471. Further, the property capital accounts (Note 20), show that the surgery is owned by four out of the six partners: Drs Black, White, Green and Brown. Note 15 (page 107) specifies that the surplus on the property income and expenditure during the year (£2100) must be appropriated only to those four partners as joint owners. Profits from this source are allocated between the four partners by crediting £525 to each of them (Note 2, page 102).

10 *Prior shares of profit.* Many practices have arrangements in force so that particular items of income are allocated between the partners in different ratios to the main practice profits. Note 2 refers to this prin-ciple as applying to: net surgery income; night visit fees; seniority awards; and the postgraduate education allowance. The partners have, in this case, agreed to retain their night visit fees, which have been allocated in the exact proportions in which they were earned; seniority and PGEA has been allocated on a similar basis, so that out of the total profit realized (£348 633), a total of £34 236 is extracted before the remaining profits are allocated between the partners in agreed ratios.

11 *GP fundholding.* Note 14 indicates that this is a fundholding practice, and sets out the amounts received under the management allowance, as well as how it is allocated to various items of expenditure.

The summary income and expenditure account shows the expenses and refunds of a non-capital nature (£31 429) on both sides of the accounts, as items of income and expenditure, in order to avoid 'netting out' (*see* below).

Part of the management allowance (£3071) has been spent on capital assets.

12 *'Grossing up'*. The details of income and expenditure (Notes 10 and 13) show that all expenses for which refunds are wholly or partially received (*see* Chapter 10) have been properly and fully grossed up. By this means, the accounts show the maximum level of expenditure in case of selection in the Review Body sampling process. This process has been applied in these accounts to: dispensing drugs; rates and water; ancillary staff salaries; trainees' salaries; and the fundholding management allowance.

13 *Current accounts*. The partners' current accounts on page 111 are, in effect, their bank accounts with the practice. They give details of the profits earned by each partner and any additional credits, such as leave advances and tax repayments, and of the manner in which they have been paid out, in terms of drawings, superannuation, national insurance, income tax, etc.

   The final balances, provided that adequate funds have been set aside to provide for a working capital requirement, represent the undrawn profits of the partners, and can be withdrawn by them once the accounts have been approved and signed by all the partners. Failure to operate this equalization procedure each year will almost certainly result in a 'snowball' effect, with the disparity between the partners' current account balances increasing steadily until it reaches an unacceptable level.

14 *Drawings*. Page 112 represents the cash withdrawals from the practice by the partners. Drawings are payments on account of the profits being earned by the partners (*see* Chapter 26). It is impossible for these to be calculated accurately during the year, hence the need for the equalization procedure outlined above. Nevertheless, it is helpful if a schedule of such drawings can be included in the accounts, so that the partners can check these figures against their own records.

The practice manager should, in an enlightened and forward-looking practice, be made familiar with the practice accounts. In many partnerships, a separate set of the accounts are made available for her and she is expected to discuss them with the partners. The practice manager should also be invited to any meetings with the accountant.

It is normal for accounts, when completed and agreed by the partners, to be signed by them—a space in the accounts has been provided for these signatures on page 98. Signature of annual accounts is normally provided for in partnership deeds.

DRS BLACK, WHITE, GREEN, BROWN, ORANGE AND GREY
PARTNERSHIP ACCOUNTS
YEAR ENDED 30 JUNE 1993

Contents

Note The above page references are to pages in this book. In practice, pages 201 and 236 would be included within the statement of accounts, but are shown separately here for information purposes only.

DRS BLACK, WHITE, GREEN, BROWN, ORANGE AND GREY
ACCOUNTANTS' REPORT
YEAR ENDED 30 JUNE 1993

We have prepared the accounts for the year ended 30 June 1993 on records produced to us and from information and explanations given to us.

We have not carried out an audit.

TICK, FIDDLE & POST
Chartered Accountants

BRANCASTER
25 September 1993

CONFIRMATION BY THE PARTNERS

We approve these accounts and confirm that the accounting records produced, together with information and explanations supplied to Tick, Fiddle & Post constitute a true and correct record of all the transactions of this practice for the year ended 30 June 1993.

....
Dr J W T Black

....
Dr D M White

....
Dr W J Green

....
Dr S J Brown

....
Dr M Orange

....
Dr A C Grey

DRS BLACK, WHITE, GREEN, BROWN, ORANGE AND GREY
DISTRIBUTION OF PROFIT
YEAR ENDED 30 JUNE 1993

	Page	1993 £	1992 £
Income	100	618 175	518 121
Expenditure	100	270 788	194 739
		347 387	323 382
Investment income	100	1246	847
Net profit		348 633	324 229

Allocated as follows:

	Prior shares (Note 2) £	Share of balance (Note 3) £	1993 total £	1992 total £
Dr Black	6279	37 466	43 745	69 752
Dr White	9374	66 286	75 660	71 946
Dr Green	6524	66 286	72 810	68 347
Dr Brown	5597	66 286	71 883	67 246
Dr Orange	5187	62 354	67 541	46 938
Dr Grey	1275	15 719	16 994	–
	34 236	314 397	348 633	324 229

DRS BLACK, WHITE, GREEN, BROWN, ORANGE AND GREY
INCOME AND EXPENDITURE ACCOUNT
YEAR ENDED 30 JUNE 1993

	Notes	1993 £	£	1992 £	£
Income:					
National Health Service fees	4	317 380		299 925	
Dispensing fees	9	3462		2546	
Reimbursements	10	191 960		182 797	
Appointments	11	61 466		19 428	
Other fees	12	12 478		13 425	
Fundholding management allowance	14	31 429		–	
Total income			618 175		518 121
Expenditure:					
Practice expenses	13	44 695		47 877	
Premises expenses	13	17 447		12 762	
Staff expenses	13	123 462		73 422	
Administration expenses	13	8270		7254	
Financial expenses	13	41 539		51 077	
Depreciation	17	3946		2347	
Fundholding expenses	14	31 429		–	
Total expenditure			270 788		194 739
			347 387		323 382
Investment income:					
Building society interest			1246		847
Net profit for the year (page 99)			348 633		324 229

DRS BLACK, WHITE, GREEN, BROWN, ORANGE AND GREY
BALANCE SHEET
YEAR ENDED 30 JUNE 1993

	Notes	1993 £	1993 £	1992 £	1992 £
Partners' funds and reserves:					
Property capital accounts	20		202 225		199 170
Capital accounts	21		80 000		60 000
Current accounts	22		5852		4364
			288 077		263 534
Employment of funds:					
Surgery premises	16		631 471		627 524
Fixed assets	17		59 264		48 925
Current assets:					
Stock of drugs		4275		3940	
Debtors		12 946		13 869	
Balance at building society		6492		9421	
Cash at bank and in hand		12 465		232	
		36 178		27 462	
Current liabilities:					
Bank overdraft		–		3450	
Creditors		8642		7828	
Due to former partner	19	948		745	
		9590		12 023	
Net current assets			26 588		15 439
Net assets			717 323		691 888
Long-term liabilities:					
Property mortgage	18		429 246		428 354
Net assets			288 077		263 534

DRS BLACK, WHITE, GREEN, BROWN, ORANGE AND GREY
NOTES TO THE ACCOUNTS
YEAR ENDED 30 JUNE 1993

1   Accounting policies

1.1   The income and expenditure account is prepared so as to reflect actual income earned, and expenditure incurred, during the year.

1.2   The stock of drugs is valued at the lower of cost or net realizable value.

1.3   Fixed assets are written off over their estimated useful lives. The following rates of depreciation are applied to the assets in use at the balance sheet date:

Furniture and fittings	– 10% per annum on cost
Computer equipment	– 33⅓% per annum on cost or book value
Office and medical equipment	– 20% per annum on cost or book value

The surgery premises are not depreciated.

1.4   The income and expenditure for the year has been allocated between the periods shown in Note 3 on the time apportionment basis.

1.5   The accounts are prepared taking into account principles outlined in the General Medical Services Statement of Fees and Allowances.

2   Prior shares of profit

	Night visit fees	Seniority	PGEA	Net surgery income (Note 15)	Total
	£	£	£	£	£
Dr Black	1948	2625	1181	525	6279
Dr White	2264	4541	2044	525	9374
Dr Green	1846	2109	2044	525	6524
Dr Brown	2624	404	2044	525	5597
Dr Orange	3143	–	2044	–	5187
Dr Grey	412	–	863	–	1275
	12 237	9679	10 220	2100	34 236

DRS BLACK, WHITE, GREEN, BROWN, ORANGE AND GREY
NOTES TO THE ACCOUNTS (continued)
YEAR ENDED 30 JUNE 1993

3 Distribution of profit

	Period to 30 Sept 1992 %	Period to 31 Jan 1993 %	Period to 30 June 1993 %
Dr Black	21	20	–
Dr White	21	20	22
Dr Green	21	20	22
Dr Brown	21	20	22
Dr Orange	16	20	22
Dr Grey	–	–	12
	100	100	100

Share of balance:

	£	£	£	Total £
Dr Black	16 506	20 960	–	37 466
Dr White	16 506	20 960	28 820	66 286
Dr Green	16 506	20 960	28 820	66 286
Dr Brown	16 506	20 960	28 820	66 286
Dr Orange	12 575	20 959	28 820	62 354
Dr Grey	–	–	15 719	15 719
	78 599	104 799	130 999	314 397

4 National Health Service fees

	Note	1993 £	1992 £
Practice allowances, etc	5	61 060	59 262
Capitation fees	6	193 602	182 015
Sessional fees	7	16 691	18 250
Item of service fees	8	46 027	40 398
		317 380	299 925

5 Practice allowances, etc

	1993	1992
Practice allowances	32 220	30 802
Seniority awards	9670	9200
Postgraduate education allowances	10 220	10 625
Rural practice payments	4670	4395
Trainee supervision grant	4280	4240
	61 060	59 262

DRS BLACK, WHITE, GREEN, BROWN, ORANGE AND GREY
NOTES TO THE ACCOUNTS (continued)
YEAR ENDED 30 JUNE 1993

6 Capitation

	1993 £	1992 £
Capitation fees	143 400	137 664
Registration fees	8700	8500
Child health surveillance fees	6250	5938
Deprivation payments	4600	4200
Target payments:		
Cervical cytology	7850	6305
Childhood immunizations	9462	7462
Pre-school boosters	13 340	11 946
	193 602	182 015

7 Sessional payments

Health promotion clinics	12 145	13 008
Minor surgery	2746	2462
Medical students	1800	2780
	16 691	18 250

8 Item of service fees

Night visits	12 237	9862
Temporary residents	6162	7871
Contraceptive services	8700	5879
Emergency treatment and INT	191	284
Maternity	12 619	10 716
Vaccinations and immunizations	6118	5786
	46 027	40 398

9 Other NHS income

Dispensing fees	3462	2546

DRS BLACK, WHITE, GREEN, BROWN, ORANGE AND GREY
NOTES TO THE ACCOUNTS (continued)
YEAR ENDED 30 JUNE 1993

10 Reimbursements

	1993 £	1992 £
Premises:		
Rent	42 364	42 364
Rates and water rates	10 465	8462
Ancillary staff salaries:		
Salaries	55 246	30 561
National Insurance	5364	4648
Training	1346	–
Trainees' salary	24 680	21 240
Computer maintenance	2750	1645
Drugs	49 745	38 877
	191 960	147 797

11 Appointments

	1993 £	1992 £
Taxed Schedule E:		
Brancaster General Hospital (Dr White)	9648	8462
St John's Hospital (Dr Brown)	2645	2520
Other appointments:		
Police surgeon's fees	41 275	3246
Midworth Nursing Home	4275	3445
ABC Ltd	739	–
XYZ Ltd	1194	1755
St Peter's School	1690	–
	61 466	19 428

12 Other fees

	1993 £	1992 £
Private patients	5249	5270
Insurance examinations etc	5946	4280
Cremations	150	120
Sundry	1133	3755
	12 478	13 425

DRS BLACK, WHITE, GREEN, BROWN, ORANGE AND GREY
NOTES TO THE ACCOUNTS (continued)
YEAR ENDED 30 JUNE 1993

13 Expenditure

	1993 £	1992 £
Practice expenses:		
Drugs and instruments	37 426	35 462
Locum fees	421	3546
Relief services fees	3022	6084
Hire and maintenance of equipment	1275	843
NHS levies	462	420
Practice replacements	694	527
Medical books	750	575
Courses and conferences	645	420
	44 695	47 877
Premises expenses:		
Rates and water rates	10 465	8462
Heat and light	3469	2570
Insurance	1240	947
Maintenance and repair	1847	509
Cleaning and laundry	426	274
	17 447	12 762
Staff expenses:		
Ancillary staff salaries	89 132	44 901
Trainee salaries	24 697	21 246
Training expenses	3962	1750
Recruitment costs	425	875
Staff welfare	5246	4650
	123 462	73 422
Administration expenses:		
Postage and stationery	408	925
Telephone	2546	2296
Accountancy fees	4390	3625
Sundries	426	408
Professional fees	500	–
	8270	7254
Finance expenses:		
Bank interest and charges	1275	2380
Surgery loan interest	40 264	48 697
	41 539	51 077

DRS BLACK, WHITE, GREEN, BROWN, ORANGE AND GREY
NOTES TO THE ACCOUNTS (continued)
YEAR ENDED 30 JUNE 1993

14 Fundholding management allowance

		1993 £	1992 £
Allowance received for capital assets		3071	
Allowance received for revenue expenditure		31 429	
		34 500	
Capital expenditure:			
Photocopier	1150		
Word processor	1921	(3071)	
		31 429	
Revenue expenditure:			
Staff salaries	24 978		
Telephone	1346		
Stationery	924		
Training	1536		
Computer maintenance	1370		
Accountancy	1175		
Recruitment	100	31 429	
Net income			

15 Net surgery income/expenses

	1993	1992
Notional rent	42 364	42 364
Less: Interest	40 264	48 697
	2100	(6333)

16 Surgery premises

Freehold property:
The Medical Centre, High Street,
Brancaster

	1993	1992
At cost to 30 June 1992	627 524	627 524
Additions during year	3947	–
	631 471	627 524

DRS BLACK, WHITE, GREEN, BROWN, ORANGE AND GREY
NOTES TO THE ACCOUNTS (continued)
YEAR ENDED 30 JUNE 1993

17 Fixed assets

	Furniture & fittings £	Computer equipment £	Office & medical equipment £	Total £
Cost				
At 1 July 1992	39 178	22 496	5283	66 957
Additions during year	3724	25 934	665	30 323
Less: FHSA grants	–	(12 967)	–	(12 967)
Fundholding management allowance	(3071)	–	–	(3071)
At 30 June 1993	39 831	35 463	5948	81 242
Depreciation				
At 1 July 1992	6425	10 962	645	18 032
Charge for year	1875	1562	509	3946
At 30 June 1993	8300	12 524	1154	21 978
Net book amounts				
At 30 June 1993	31 531	22 939	4794	59 264
At 30 June 1992	32 753	11 534	4638	48 925

18 Property mortgage

The practice has a mortgage loan with Branshire Bank plc, secured on the freehold property and repayable by monthly instalments over 20 years.

The term of the mortgage remaining is 16 years, the interest rate is variable at 1.25% over base and at 30 June 1993 was 8%.

The monthly repayments at present are £4275 and the capital outstanding is as follows.

	1993 £	1992 £
Balance at 30 June 1992	428 354	436 618
Net advances (repayments) during year	892	(8264)
	429 246	428 354

DRS BLACK, WHITE, GREEN, BROWN, ORANGE AND GREY
NOTES TO THE ACCOUNTS (continued)
YEAR ENDED 30 JUNE 1993

19 Retired partners' account

	Dr H W Blue £	Dr J W T Black £
Balance at 1 July 1992	745	
Paid to Dr Blue		
Less: Withdrawn		
Other	745	
Transfer from partners' current accounts (page 111)		948

20 Property capital accounts

	1993 £	1992 £
Dr Black	50 557	49 793
Dr White	50 556	49 793
Dr Green	50 556	49 792
Dr Brown	50 556	49 792
	202 225	199 170
Represented as follows:		
Surgery premises (Note 16)	631 471	627 524
Less: Property mortgage (Note 18)	429 246	428 354
	202 225	199 170

21 Capital accounts

Dr Black	–	12 600
Dr White	17 600	12 600
Dr Green	17 600	12 600
Dr Brown	17 600	12 600
Dr Orange	17 600	9600
Dr Grey	9600	–
	80 000	60 000

DRS BLACK, WHITE, GREEN, BROWN, ORANGE AND GREY
NOTES TO THE ACCOUNTS (continued)
YEAR ENDED 30 JUNE 1993

	1993 £	1992 £
22 Current accounts (page 111)		
Dr Black	–	(927)
Dr White	2091	1276
Dr Green	1233	1705
Dr Brown	1648	1466
Dr Orange	1346	844
Dr Grey	(466)	–
	5852	4364

DRS BLACK, WHITE, GREEN, BROWN, ORANGE AND GREY
PARTNERS' CURRENT ACCOUNT   YEAR ENDED 30 JUNE 1993

	Total		Dr Black		Dr White		Dr Green		Dr Brown		Dr Orange		Dr Grey	
	£	£	£	£	£	£	£	£	£	£	£	£	£	£
Balances at 1 July 1992		4364		(927)		1276		1705		1466		844		–
Profit for the year (page 99)	348 633		43 745		75 660		72 810		71 883		67 541		16 994	
Leave advances	6625		–		1325		1325		1325		1325		1325	
Income tax repayment: 1991/92	5668		2746		1327		842		753		–		–	
Cash introduced	9000		–		–		–		–		–		9000	
	369 926	374 290	46 491	45 564	78 312	79 588	74 977	76 682	73 961	75 427	68 866	69 710		27 319
Less: partnership drawings														
Partners' monthly drawings (page 112)	260 029		41 523		53 139		52 558		48 027		51 228		13 554	
Superannuation:														
Standard	12 568		1466		2564		2564		2564		2193		1217	
Added years	7765		–		–		3529		4236		–		–	
On appointments	738		–		579		–		159		–		–	
Leave advances repaid	6445		958		1289		1289		1289		1289		331	
Income tax paid:														
1991/92	128		–		–		–		10 227		128		–	
1992/93	49 634		12 345		9387		9465		995		5246		2964	
PAYE tax on appointments	4623		–		3628		–		–		–		–	
National Insurance: Class 1	1106		–		868		–		238		–		–	
Class 2	1399		160		280		280		280		280		119	
	344 435	29 855	56 452	(10 888)	71 734	7854	69 685	6997	68 015	7412	60 364	9346	18 185	9134
Transfers from property capital accounts (Note 20)	(3055)		(764)		(763)		(764)		(764)		–		–	
Transfers to capital accounts (Note 21)	(20 000)		12 600		(5000)		(5000)		(5000)		(8000)		(9600)	
Transfer to retired partner's account (Note 19)	(948)		(948)		–		–		–		–		–	
		(24 003)		10 888		(5763)		(5764)		(5764)		(8000)		(9600)
Balances at 30 June 1993		5852		–		2091		1233		1648		1346		(466)

DRS BLACK, WHITE, GREEN, BROWN, ORANGE AND GREY
PARTNERS' MONTHLY DRAWINGS
YEAR ENDED 30 JUNE 1993

		£	Dr Black £	Dr White £	Dr Green £	Dr Brown £	Dr Orange £	Dr Grey £
1992	July		3000	3000	3000	3000	2300	–
	August		3000	3000	3000	3000	2300	–
	September		4352	3946	3564	3294	4784	–
	October		3500	3500	3500	3500	2700	–
	November		3500	3500	3500	3500	2700	–
	December		5325	5125	4928	4265	5027	–
	(T)		2746	1327	842	753	–	–
1993	January		3500	3500	3500	3500	2700	–
	(C)		12 600	–	–	–	–	–
	February		–	3500	3500	3500	3500	1700
	March		–	6425	6274	5947	8247	3926
	April		–	3800	3800	3800	3800	1800
	May		–	3800	3800	3800	3800	1800
	June		–	8716	9350	6168	9370	4328
		260 029	41 523	53 139	52 558	48 027	51 228	13 554

(C) Capital payment on retirement
(T) Tax payment or repayment

19 Financial Statistics

AN advantage of medical practice, which is not readily available to other businesses, is easy access to statistics that the GPs and their manager can use to judge the profitability and efficiency of the practice. Some of these are set out below.

1 *Expenditure levels.* By the averaging process, and for superannuation purposes, the DoH considers that the expenses of a medical practice currently run at about 35% of gross income. This is very low when one considers that this takes into account all items paid personally by the partners, including motoring and house expenses, and spouses' salaries, etc. It is to the GP's advantage that expenses be maximized, which can only be done by means of accounts drawn up in a manner that maximizes the income and expenses of the practice (*see* Chapter 3).

2 *Proportions of NHS income.* Figures currently available suggest that average proportions of NHS income received by a typical medical practice during 1992/93, would be as follows:

	%
Practice allowances	17
Capitation fees	63
Item of service fees	16
Sessional fees	4
	100

3 *Item of service fees.* A number of figures are available to give averages of item of service fees earned by medical practices in recent years. One of these gives the following as the average earnings of item of service fees per patient. This information is extremely valuable in attempting to evaluate the earnings of a practice.

	Return per patient			
	England	*Wales*	*Scotland*	*Northern Ireland*
Night visits	118.9p	178.4p	161.4p	198.7p
Temporary residents	34.4p	47.1p	34.4p	19.8p
Contraceptive services	91.0p	80.1p	80.0p	71.2p
Emergency treatment	3.9p	5.3p	7.8p	4.6p
Maternity medical services	142.8p	133.8p	123.9p	149.6p
Vaccinations/immunizations	56.7p	40.5p	43.3p	38.4p

Calculated from figures supplied by health departments for 1992/93.

It is possible to further evaluate the financial efficiency of the practice by comparing gross and net income levels, both on a partner and per patient basis. This is done by extracting figures from those published regularly in respect of intended average remuneration levels. These figures are already available up to March 1994, although where year-ends other than March are used, as is increasingly the case, they must be apportioned accordingly. The figures set out below show the averages for three year-ends: to March 1993, June 1993 and March 1994 (England only).

	March 1993 £	June 1993 £	March 1994 £
Gross intended remuneration:			
per principal	59 977	60 559	62 303
per patient	30.50	30.80	31.69
Net intended remuneration:			
per principal	39 977	40 011	40 113
per patient	20.33	20.35	20.40

A practice wishing to 'test' itself against the statistics for gross remuneration must therefore take into account its gross income from all fees and allowances (excluding refunds and income from non-FHSA sources), and divide this between the number of partners or the total list size as applicable.

To arrive at the figure of net remuneration, for comparison purposes, it is necessary to take all income from NHS sources, including refunds, and deduct from this the total expenditure of the practice, except expenses specifically relating to non-NHS income sources. The resulting figure should then be divided between the number of full-time partners, normally defined as those who are receiving the full rate of BPA.

4 *Other income.* Figures are available which show average returns from various other NHS income sources for the year to March 1993.

	Return per patient			
	England	*Wales*	*Scotland*	*Northern Ireland*
Health promotion	149.4p	119.6p	117.4p	56.0p
Minor surgery	46.1p	50.6p	53.3p	44.7p
Child health surveillance	41.9p	36.5p	36.9p	64.2p
New registrations	38.3p	32.9p	33.0p	21.3p

A case study

Reference to the accounts in Chapter 18 on pages 98–112 shows a set of typical GP partnership accounts which, although not bearing direct relation to any known practice, nevertheless gives statistics of the type GPs require in order to assess the financial performance of their practices, and subsequently to make management decisions and institute necessary economies. Figure 19.1 reproduces some statistics from these accounts.

The GP or practice manager interpreting these accounts has the following valuable items of information at his disposal.

1 The practice has five constant, full-time equity *partners*, and the average patient list is 1912. Gross NHS income, both per partner and per patient, is comfortably above both the previous year's performance and the intended average.

2 Net *NHS remuneration*, at £54 689 per partner and £28.6 per patient, is also well above intended averages. However, the allocation of gross NHS income shows capitation fees slightly below average, which reflects a slightly lower than average list size.

   Although net remuneration remains well above average, some concern might be felt at the drop from £58 106 per partner and £30.6 per patient in the previous year, in spite of a continued rise in gross income. This is clearly due to the rise in expenses from 33.1% to 40.2% of total income. The practice should therefore consider ways in which economies might be made.

3 The total return from *item of service fees* over the year was £4.83 per patient, which is again an improvement both on the previous year and published averages. At 15% of net NHS remuneration, they nevertheless represent a smaller than average proportion of income.

4 The return from *ancillary staff reimbursement* (68%) is below average and shows a fall from the 72% achieved in the previous year. This may be due to the imposition of cash limiting, but steps should be taken to see if this recovery rate can be improved.

5 The return from *night visit fees* has increased significantly compared with the previous year, and is now above average. Taken with the fall in deputizing and locum fee costs, this shows that the partners are performing their own night visits and receiving the higher fee, which has had a significant effect on profitability.

DRS BLACK, WHITE, GREEN, BROWN, ORANGE AND GREY
STATISTICS FOR YEAR ENDED 30 JUNE 1993

	National average 1992/93	Year ended 1993	1992
1 Average patient numbers:			
0–64	8295	7910	7868
65–74	855	920	915
75 and over	680	730	700
	9830	9560	9483
2 Average number of full-time equity partners	5	5	5
3 Average patients per partner	1966	1912	1897

	Intended income £	£	£
4 Gross NHS income (excluding reimbursements):			
per full partner	60 559	63 476	59 985
per patient	30.80	33.20	31.62
5 Net NHS income:			
per full partner	40 011	54 689	58 106
per patient	20.35	28.60	30.63

	%	%	%
6 Allocation of gross NHS income:			
Practice allowances	17	19	20
Capitation fees	63	61	61
Sessional fees	4	5	6
Item of service fees	16	15	13
	100	100	100

	National average 1991/92 £	£	£
7 Item of service income per patient:			
Night visits	1.20	1.28	1.04
Temporary residents	0.33	0.64	0.83
Contraceptive services	0.87	0.91	0.62
Emergency treatment and INT	0.04	0.02	0.03
Maternity	1.37	1.32	1.13
Vaccinations and immunizations	0.49	0.64	0.61
	4.30	4.81	4.26
8 Ancillary staff reimbursements	–	68%	72%
9 Expense/earnings ratio	–	40.2%	33.1%

Figure 19.1   Statistics extracted from a specimen set of accounts (*see* pages 98–112)

20 The Use of Computers

The direct reimbursement scheme

INVESTMENT in computers in general practice is probably the third largest capital expense (after premises and cars). It is estimated that GPs will spend £56 million on bespoke medical computer systems in 1993. That is nearly £2000 for every principal. Much of this is financed by a government direct reimbursement scheme, the rules of which remain unchanged until April 1994 and are specified in paragraph 58 of the SFA.

The scale of reimbursement is shown in Table 20.1 and is based on practice list size.

Table 20.1 Scale for direct reimbursement of practice computer costs

List size	Purchase £	Lease £	Maintenance £	Staff £
1–2000	1800	450	270	490
2001–4000	2410	600	360	600
4001–6000	2900	720	440	770
6001–8000	3400	850	510	840
8001–10 000	4200	1050	630	900
10 001–12 000	5500	1370	830	970
12 001–14 000	6000	1500	900	1030
14 001–16 000	6500	1620	980	1090
16 001–18 000	7000	1750	1050	1160
18 001–20 000	7500	1870	1130	1240

These scales are a guide for FHSAs; they are not mandatory, but are subject to funds available. Up to 50% of the cost and maintenance of an eligible system may be reimbursed.

Fundholders, however, may be reimbursed 100% of fund-holding software and 75% of hardware costs. Since the funds are cash-limited, there is then little left in FHSA coffers for others. It is not possible to estimate the chances of a non-fundholder attracting funds since local preferences vary.

It is essential to remain on good terms with the local computer FHSA facilitator and finance director. Prepare a business plan early in the NHS financial year (starting 1 April) when making a bid—your gain is bound to be at the expense of another practice. Before committing the practice to buying or enhancing a computer system, you should obtain a written commitment from the FHSA as to the funds they have allocated to your practice for reimbursement, and the length of time that this offer remains open.

Many GPs have become disenchanted because reimbursements allegedly promised are not honoured, leaving the doctors with a large bill and no government grant. This situation may arise due to a genuine misunderstanding by either party or because the FHSA has run out of cash, possibly due to a later, fundholding applicant taking priority.

Towards the end of the NHS financial year, it is just possible that computer reimbursement funds have not been exhausted, due to another practice deferring or abandoning its plans, or because an unexpected top-up has been received from the RHA. A telephone call to the finance department or FHSA computer facilitator should determine the position.

New standards and developments

In 1992, the DoH commissioned a study to determine a Minimum System Specification for GP computers. This report went through a metamorphosis as Activity Analysis in General Practice (AAGP) and emerged as Requirements for Accreditation for GP Computer Systems.

GP computer suppliers will be expected to deliver systems with modules that conform to such specifications, although not every practice will choose at first to acquire or upgrade a system that covers every activity. However, the ruling ensures an agreed common standard of upgrade, so that no doctor will in future hit a dead end if the supplier goes out of business as the investment in data entry will not be wasted. Target date for implementation of the standard is April 1994. GPs who own systems whose suppliers do not offer this upgrade path are unlikely to receive any reimbursement from their FHSA after 31 March 1994.

A criticism of Requirements for Accreditation is that the NHS management executive have set up an unnecessarily complicated administrative protocol for the scheme, and insisted on unnecessarily complex and expensive software. It is alleged that maternity claims have over 130 stipulations for payment.

The NHS is developing a National Health Service Administrative Register (NHSAR). Every patient will be issued with a new nine-figure NHS number. At present only the central registry at Stockport is electronically linked with all FHSAs. At last, most duplicate patients have been weeded out, and a common address and personal details agreed, but these particulars may not be up to date. The next stage is to merge the RHA and FHSA registers to create regional NHS administrative registers. This should facilitate better planning, delivery and audit of health care.

Pilot schemes linking general practices electronically with FHSAs are proceeding. Registration data exchange between practices and the FHSAs has been successful and is being extended to electronic submission of item of service fees. Ultimately a keyboard entry at the practice will send a claim to the FHSA which will be electronically validated and then manually re-appraised at the practice source. Such a system will be electronically linked to the GP's quarterly pay statement and the money sent to his bank through the clearing system network (BACS).

Ultimately, when a patient moves, marries, dies or changes sex, a key-board entry at the practice will change the details on the central computers. This will call for a high degree of GP staff education, training and discipline, as well as tight controls to ensure confidentiality. An erroneous entry at any terminal on the NHS network could degrade the quality of data.

System specifications

To qualify for reimbursement for the NHS year beginning 1 April 1994, the GP computer system must conform to the following requirements.

- Transfer of data possible in simple 'text file' format.
- An audit trail showing the date, time, and 'author' of every entry and revision. This feature enables a reconstruction of a record as it was at any given time in the past, which is useful for medico-legal purposes; it 'stops the clock' and allows an assessment of the data available at the time, putting aside the benefit of hindsight.
- Use of Read five figure codes for diagnoses.
- A drug dictionary and brand/generic comparisons of costs.
- Standardization of FHSA/GP and health net link protocols.
- Item of service claims possible by electronic data interchange.
- Fund-holding protocol links.
- Standard search routines.
- Back-up procedures with less than 15 minutes' continuous operator super-vision (multiple floppy disk back-up does not qualify).
- A computer supplier helpline response and maintenance support con-forming to defined acceptable response times.

In order to meet these criteria, the main central processor unit needs to be at least of fast 486 calibre, the hard disc capacity at least 100MB, and the on board memory will need to be expanded. The back-up medium should be a tape streamer or other storage device.

Practice requirements and expenses

The computer will need a physical lock on the system box and the computer room must have a robust lock.

Since the required product will be a major system modification, all equipment attached to it will need to conform to the EEC standards which came into force for new equipment on 1 January 1993. The keyboard must be detachable, the monitor should tilt and swivel, and conform to radiation standards, and all equipment attached to it should be comfortably accessible to the operator.

The computer operator must be housed in a temperature controlled environment with adequate working space. Clerks must no longer be required to work in airless, hot cubby holes. Processor boxes tucked under a shelf or noisy printers, positioned close to workers, with replacement of paper requiring the agility of a gymnast, are not acceptable.

Although the price of hardware has come down, the upgrading of terminals and other equipment is itself a costly exercise. Consideration must also be given to expanding the physical space; otherwise the practice may fail an inspection by the Environmental Health Officer, as well as failing to care properly for its employees' working environment.

Second-hand equipment has a very low value but, provided it conforms to the standards, your present kit may prove suitable to run stand-alone word processing or spreadsheet calculations.

Remember that all computer equipment must conform to the EEC safety standards by 1 January 1996. Already the chairs of all staff using terminals must be of adjustable height with a foot rest, if required, and with a movable back rest; the desk-top work space must not be cramped, so that there is room for all relevant paperwork and materials, and an adjustable document holder if necessary; and the screen must be positioned to avoid reflections.

Screen burn, caused by the VDU glass becoming etched with a constant image such as the menu command line, may blur the screen and is unacceptable. This is avoided by installing a software screen saver, so that after a short time of no keyboard activity the screen goes blank or may be replaced by moving images, such as fish in an aquarium. A rapid 'time out' of the screen saver is essential in areas to which patients have access, in order to safeguard confidentiality and conform to the Data Protection Act.

Both the hardware and improvements to the working environment are bound to be costly; the practice manager and the computer supplier should both make a detailed and careful inventory of all kit on site.

In addition, the software is likely to need a major rewrite, and in some cases a change of operating system. Software design and debugging is a labour intensive and expensive process. However, if the practice's supplier has a large user base, the cost may be spread across 500 or more general practice customers.

Some companies are quoting for software development at 1–2 million pounds per annum, including substantial accreditation fees which must be borne by the supplier. Maintenance costs just to cope with item of service and target changes, and the flexible interpretation of the rules by different FHSAs, are substantial. Assuming a user base of 500 systems, the minimum software charge will be £2000 per system before any profit is taken. However, there are about 15 companies with a user base of 100 or more GP customers. If their present systems are of recent design and the software is robust, they could achieve accreditation at modest cost, particularly if the GP system is not their only product.

Practices which have bought a system with few existing users are likely to be forced to migrate. The key to changing systems is the portability of data. It is likely that the basic registration features of name, address, DOB and NHS number will not be a problem. Should a user group migrate en masse, then it is likely that, with the co-operation of the original supplier and disclosure of source codes, much of the other data can be taken across too, albeit at a price. Piecemeal change of users to different suppliers is likely to leave the abandoned systems as data cemeteries, in which case a paper print-out of each patient's details must be kept in their medical record envelope. Some facilitators would argue that, in this situation, a mass decision would generally be made to change supplier.

Computer hardware depreciates over a three to five year period, which must be allowed for in a practice business plan. Software needs constant maintenance. It is unwise to purchase software and hardware from different suppliers. It is essential to have a maintenance contract for the main CPU and terminals, but printers are robust and you may choose to forgo a maintenance contract for them as, in the long run, it may be cheaper either to pay for repairs or buy a new printer if necessary. When replacing a noisy dot matrix printer, it is worth considering a quieter model, such as an ink jet printer, for use in the consulting room.

Database value for the team

The usefulness of a well maintained database, in terms of administration and enhanced patient care, outweighs the disadvantage of high depreciation. Table 20.2 illustrates the value of accumulating and maintaining good data. This table is derived from a spreadsheet: the first column shows the occupations of practice team members; the second column shows the hourly rates of gross pay; and the other columns estimate likely amounts of time spent on, and the value of, database entries (as a percentage and in pounds) per member(s) of staff engaged in each occupation.

There can be little argument that the computing activity of repeat prescription and fund-holding clerks has a value of 100%. The nurse may seem to have a surprisingly high data entry value. This is because, although much of her work is hands on care of patients, the added value of certain services she carries out may bring in, either directly or indirectly, substantial cash sums. All immunizations contribute towards achievements of targets or item of service payments, cervical cytology has a high target award and helping with minor surgery generates payments. It is essential that there is a terminal in every treatment room and nursing station. Ideally the nurse should make the keyboard entry herself at the time the treatment is given. Deferred entries often fail to be recorded and are prone to error; it is far easier to call up the patient's computer record on the spot. This allows recording of extra events such as smoking habits when the patient is present, and painlessly accumulates information for health promotion banding claims.

Receptionists often have the local knowledge to verify changes of address, confirm telephone numbers and input new registrations. They should each have a terminal—a good rule of thumb is that there should be one at every telephone point.

The value of a GP's time in relation to the value of his data input is a much debated issue. He may wish to change the figures and look at the result.

In the example (Table 20.2), a total data value of nearly £3000 a week is suggested (£149 523 a year). However, this is difficult to sustain: 25% of this figure, ie £37 381 pa or £3.12 for each patient record, is probably more realistic.

Safeguarding the system

It is essential that this valuable resource is safeguarded. Back-ups must be carried out daily, but not during normal working hours (if the system is down and patients are being seen their data will not be properly entered).

Table 20.2 Estimated value of the database per job title in a six-doctor practice with a list size of 12 000

	hourly rate of pay (£)	hours/day	days/week	hours/week	Data value as % of time	Data value/week (£)	Possible* data value/year (£)
Receptionists	4.24	21.0	5.0	105.0	25	111	5565
Repeat prescription clerks	4.24	20.0	5.0	100.0	100	424	21 200
Secretary	4.40	4.0	5.0	20.0	20	18	880
Practice manager	10.00	8.0	5.0	40.0	40	160	8000
Clerks	4.24	10.0	5.0	50.0	50	106	5300
Administrator	7.80	8.0	5.0	40.0	40	125	6240
Nurses	8.00	15.0	5.0	75.0	90	540	27 000
Fundholding clerks	4.35	13.0	5.0	65.0	100	283	14 138
GPs	40.00	24.0	5.1	122.4	25	1224	61 200
Totals		168		622		2990	149 523

* The annual totals from this example are unrealistic. For a practice of this size a notional value per year might be 25% of the total or £37 381 pa. This would be a data value per patient of £3.12 pa.

At least three back-up copies should be kept in a secure, magnetic, dust and damp free place, preferably in a fireproof safe in a different room to the main processor. One copy must be kept off site and an archive copy retained once a month.

It is imperative that back-ups are tested from time to time, otherwise a false sense of security may be built up, but *never* test a back up on your own computer. It should always be loaded and restored on another spare computer. Your supplier should be able to check the back-up disk(s) or tape for integrity. No amount of insurance can reinstate your previous data if a clean back-up is not available, and insurance claims are usually conditional on a proper back-up having been made.

The computer systems administrator

Every practice should have a computer systems administrator, usually an existing member of staff who may have a particular interest in the system. He or she should have a written job description which should include the tasks listed in Box 20.1.

Box 20.1: Job description for a computer systems administrator

- Take responsibility for day to day administration of the system.
- Report faults and difficulties found by other members of staff. If simple, correct; otherwise call supplier's help desk.
- Keep log of all back-ups, help desk calls and error messages.
- Liaise with supplier's engineers. Make at least two extra back-ups before engineers call for routine upgrading.
- Read and comply with suppliers' notices.
- Install user upgrades and test system.
- Check supplies of disks, tapes, consumables and paper (running out of FP10 comp is disastrous).

Security and confidentiality:
- Supervise a regular change of passwords, particularly when a member of staff leaves.
- Check Data Protection Act registration. The fee of £75 is valid for three years. Failure to register is a criminal offence: maximum penalty £5000.

Box 20.1: *continued*

- Check that terminals conform to the Act and cannot be seen by the public.
- Check that unauthorized software is not used (invalidates warranty; virus risk).
- Mark with post code all computer kit and other machines, such as faxes.
- Make an inventory of all hardware and software with registration numbers, approximate value and date purchased.
- Check that *all* practice BT lines are registered for free total care with a four-hour response.
- Check that faxes have correct title headers and adjust times at summer/ winter change.
- Check that all printouts are shredded.
- Ensure that computer prescription paper is kept in a secure place.
- Check that all work stations and furniture comply with EEC regulations.
- Ensure that eye tests are offered to all VDU operators and that spectacles are paid for by the employer.
- Liaise with suppliers at all times.
- Attend supplier courses and schemes run by other agencies and user groups.
- Induct all new recruits, including locums to the practice, on keyboard skills and protocols.
- Arrange for in-house or external courses for staff. Whilst most practice staff will already have keyboard skills, the doctors may not and will appreciate simple typing tuition.
- Emphasize the importance of confidentiality and protection of security of the system, infringement of which is a sackable offence.

The systems administrator usually reports to the practice manager, who should carry out spot checks from time to time. An enhancement of salary is appropriate to reflect the responsibility.

Accounting packages

In addition to the clinical system, there may be a fundholding accounting system. This might be integrated with the clinical system or function on a 'stand alone' basis. The supplier may have their own or a recommended business system which is coupled with the clinical system.

There are a variety of accounting and payroll systems which may be industry standard or which have been adapted for GP purposes. The Ferguson package is simple and the Sage payroll system is constantly updated. In all cases, you should ask the supplier for the names of local users and, if possible, these practices should be visited.

Of vital importance is the time taken to train staff to familiarize themselves with the package and enter data. This will reap dividends when staff time is later saved and tasks are carried out efficiently in-house rather than by an outside agency. Remember that, in most cases, GP staff are subsidized, whereas an accountant has to add 17.5% VAT to all bills as well as a profit margin. In every case where loan finance is involved, purchases should be discussed with the practice accountant.

The software spreadsheet is a useful tool. It is a piece of electronic graph paper whose cells are full of calculation magic: budgets, cash flows and staff rotas can easily be constructed with a minimum of training, and changing a figure in one cell can compute a 'what if' calculation in a series of dependent cells. The tables in this chapter have been made on a spreadsheet. Your local computer supplier should have a demonstration disk which you can use either at the computer store or run on your personal (not practice) computer system.

It is possible, but not always recommended, to run your accounts on a spreadsheet, provided the module is simple and well constructed, and with locked protected areas. It is inadvisable for more than one person to have access to such a template, as cell values may be accidentally changed. Again, always check with your accountant. There are no common standards for the nomenclature of GP fees and allowances and your accountant's in-house computer probably has a rigid structure whose software may not lend itself to use in general practice.

The Financial Special Interest Group, of the Primary Health Care Group (part of the British Computer Society), has set up a working party to look at the integration of all aspects of GP accounting. The missing links in the planned chain are the practice/accountant 'electronic hooks'. Ideally these should complete the circular reference of generating a standard framework of practice accounts that can be presented to the practice partners, passed on to the tax inspector (and, if necessary, the Inland Revenue, to sample expenses), and the results passed to the Review Body, to accurately reimburse expenses. This assumes that the Doctors' and Dentists' Review Body mechanism remains in place.

Box 20.2: How to computerize the practice—a summary

1 Consult your local FHSA or regional computer facilitator. They are of varying quality and experience, but should be able to put you in touch with both suppliers and other practices, who could be using the kit that would suit you.

2 Attend exhibitions of GP computer suppliers. Having narrowed down the field, invite up to three suppliers to give a demonstration at your premises or a partner's house. Protect the time allocated to these demonstrations; it is neither fair to the supplier nor to yourselves to have constant interruptions. Make sure that key staff who will use the system are free to come.

3 All computer training sessions should be looked upon as an investment. A day's on site training costs about £350 including VAT; add to this the hourly cost of your staff attending and it can total £100 an hour. A late start or staff popping in and out cause a loss of concentration of the trainer and students and a valuable, structured exercise is thus wasted. Follow-up staged training is equally important. Remember the potential value of your data, and that it will not be realized unless the staff are properly educated and trained.

Useful addresses

Primary Health Care Specialist Group
British Computer Society
First Floor
30 Barbourne Road
Worcester
WR1 1HT
Tel: 0905 619010
Fax: 0905 617539

Data Protection Registrar
Springfield House
Water Lane
Wilmslow
Cheshire
SK9 5AX
Tel: 0625 535777

Computer facilitators: your FHSA and the Primary Health Care Group keep a list.

Dr Bob Bowles, the author of this chapter, is a former GP and an Independent Adviser on GP Finance and Computing. He is founder Chairman of the Financial Special Interest Group, Primary Health Care Specialist Group, BCS. Tel: 0297 442100; Fax: 0297 445192.

21 The GP Partnership

THE latest available figures tell us that there are over 33 000 unrestricted GP principals practising in the United Kingdom. Of these, 81%, or about 26 000 doctors, practise as members of groups or partnerships. The vast majority are in formal partnerships, which pool profits into a common fund and divide them according to previously agreed ratios.

A business partnership has been defined as 'two or more people trading together with a view to profit'. The more whimsical have pointed out that a partnership is the most intimate form of human contact outside marriage! However, the common denominator in all GP partnerships is that they are made up of a number of doctors combining together, hopefully to their mutual advantage, who should all have a common purpose and similar direction.

All too often, partnerships founder, in some cases through the personal failings of one or more of the partners, but more often due to lack of business acumen and the absence of the true philosophy of a partnership. Many GPs who form partnerships shun co-operation and seek to go their own way: they run their own lists of patients, jealously guard their independence, and make little contact, either in the practice or personally, with their fellow partners.

The modern GP partnership should operate much as other businesses, such as solicitors', accountants' or architects' partnerships. They should: be bound by a properly drawn-up partnership deed; meet regularly to discuss common problems, both of a clinical and business nature; probably devolve the administration and management of the practice to a qualified practice manager; accept professional advice when it is proffered; and operate a common business policy, formulated by discussion and agreement.

Why do GPs form partnerships? Some GPs prefer to remain in sole practice; they may have had an unfortunate experience in partnership which has affected their outlook, or they may see a partnership as a restriction on their independence. However, the number of such GPs is diminishing and it is not difficult to envisage the end of most single-handed practices within the next 20 years or so. For the most part, GPs recognize the benefits of operating in a partnership, which are outlined in Box 21.1.

Box 21.1: Advantages and disadvantages of the GP partnership

Advantages
- Facility for discussion and referral.
- Operation of a common policy.
- Easier out-of-hours responsibility.
- Pooling of expenses: economies of scale.
- Likely increased profitability.
- Potential for tax savings (*see* Chapter 39).
- Control over succession.

Disadvantages
- Perceived loss of independence.
- Earnings for benefit of partners.

The main advantage of partnership lies in the pooling of resources. Large practices have less difficulty in covering their own out-of-hours duties, usually by operating their own rotas. This facility becomes more important with the incidence of higher fees for night visits performed within the practice's own organization. In addition, common practice offers economy in costs; for instance, a partnership of two GPs is unlikely to incur a level of practice expenses double those of a single-handed practice. The potential for tax savings available to some partnerships is discussed in Chapters 31 and 39.

Many GPs wish to control the succession to their practice. A sole practitioner who retires has no such control, whereas a partnership can introduce new partners, subject to necessary approval.

Pooling of income

Many partnerships encounter difficulties when some GPs have medical earnings from various sources which they wish to retain for their own benefit. Although this is at the discretion of the partners, who will determine their own financial policy, one usually finds that, in partnerships with the greater traditions of financial discipline, all earnings from medical sources are paid into the partnership pool for division, regardless of when and how they are earned. This is likely to be set out in a clause in the partnership deed.

The retention of medical earnings by individual partners is a major source of dissent and at times has been responsible for the break-up of partnerships.

Partnership deeds

All partnerships should have, as their internal control document, a deed of partnership, preferably drawn up by a solictor specializing in the field. This will lay down the internal constitution of the partnership and partners should be prepared to adhere to it. The draft for the deed should be perused by the practice accountant, who should be able to advise on the various financial aspects.

Partnership deeds are examined in more detail in Chapter 22.

Partnership drawings

Whilst the profits realized by a solo GP from his practice are his own and he may do with them as he wishes, in a partnership different considerations apply. All partners have a responsibility towards one another and must ensure that funds withdrawn from the practice are done so on a systematic and controlled basis.

A common feature of partnership, not only within the medical profession, is that it is virtually impossible to calculate the exact profit being earned until the annual partnership accounts are drawn up. Therefore, the partners normally withdraw funds at the end of each month for their personal use. It is essential that these are calculated in accordance with properly drawn-up principles, both to ensure equity between the partners and to avoid the need for large adjustments at the end of each year to bring the capital and current accounts into proper ratios.

The drawings of the partners are not salaries, but are merely payments on account of profits, which will be taken into consideration when the annual accounts are prepared. If it emerges that a partner has underdrawn his profits, he may be able to withdraw additional funds; if he has over-drawn, then it is reasonable to expect him to repay the difference. A typical schedule of partnership drawings for a year is set out in the partnership accounts on page 112.

A GP partner is *not* assessed for tax on drawings, but on the profits earned during any given year of account. If, for instance, a GP were to earn £40 000 in one year, but withdraw only £35 000 from the partnership, his tax assessment in the following year would be based on £40 000.

Detailed calculations with regard to systems of partnership drawings and income tax reserves are set out in Chapter 26.

Partnership capital

New partners are often required to introduce capital into the partnership. The question of partnership capital and how it is funded is considered more fully in Chapters 30 and 31.

22 Partnership Deeds

IT is a well-worn cliché to compare general medical partnership with marriage, but it is a fair comparison; the problems and traumas that arise in marriage have their counterpart in general medical partnerships. In this chapter, we discuss the need for and how to facilitate a secure and harmonious partnership arrangement as the basis for a career in general practice.

The change in working conditions and responsibility for the newly-qualified GP trainee becoming a principal and entering into partnership for the first time could hardly be more stark. He will be moving from an environment of employment on a series of fixed-term contracts, usually of six months but probably no more than 12 months, into a partnership arrangement in which he will be self-employed and which may endure for more than 30 years. During that time, a GP may expect to receive an income at today's prices in excess of 1.3 million pounds, and to be part of a partnership which will employ probably dozens of practice staff during his working life. Moreover, he will have a clear contractual responsibility for the health and care of many thousands of patients.

Many general medical partnerships have survived, apparently success-fully, without a written partnership agreement. What is the value of such a written agreement? It is argued that a verbal agreement (a 'gentleman's agreement') should suffice among professional people. It is certainly true that the law does not make any distinction between written and verbal agreements when seeking to interpret and enforce them. However, there are obvious disadvantages in not having a written agreement, since reference to a document provides better guidance regarding what has been agreed and the basis on which the partnership was established, than references to conversations, discussion, and ideas, which may have been expressed in a series of meetings over a period of many years. Where disagreements arise, the absence of a written partnership agreement can be a fundamental obstacle to settling a dispute within a general medical partnership.

The 1890 Partnership Act

Where no written or verbal agreement exists, there is statutory provision to identify the rights and duties of partners; this is to be found within the

1890 Partnership Act. The courts may in such cases look to the 1890 Act, if there is a dispute in the partnership, in order to establish rights and obligations of the partners and the terms under which the partnership should be conducted. Section 24 of the Act sets out a number of rules regarding the interests and duties of partners.

'The interests of partners in the partnership property and their rights and duties in relation to the partnership should all be determined, *subject to any agreement* expressed or implied between the partners, by the following rules.

1 All the partners are entitled to share equally in the capital and profits of the business, and must contribute equally towards the losses, whether of capital or otherwise, sustained by the firm.
2 The firm must indemnify every partner in respect of payments made and personal liabilities incurred by him:

    (a) in the ordinary and proper conduct of the business of the firm; or
    (b) in or about anything necessarily done for the preservation of the business or property of the firm.

3 A partner making, for the purpose of the partnership, any payment or advance beyond the amount of capital which he has agreed to subscribe, is entitled to interest at the rate of 5% per annum from the date of payment or advance.
4 A partner is not entitled, before the ascertainment of profits, to interest on the capital subscribed by him.
5 Every partner may take part in the management of the partnership business.
6 No partner shall be entitled to remuneration for acting in the partnership business.
7 No partner may be introduced as a partner without the consent of all existing partners.
8 Any difference arising as to ordinary matters connected with the partnership business may be decided by a majority of the partners, but no change may be made in the nature of the partnership business without the consent of all existing partners.
9 The partnership books are to be kept at the place of business of the partnership (or the principal place, if there is more than one), and every partner may, when he thinks fit, have access to and inspect and copy any of them.'

It is important to note that partners are still free, if they make a formal agreement among themselves, to depart from or amend the above rules.

Written agreements

What should a GP joining a partnership expect to find in the partnership agreement? In theory, the list could be endless, but we shall look at some of the key elements that contribute towards a sound partnership agreement and assist in creating harmony, security, and equity in general practice partnerships. It must be remembered that no written agreement will cover all eventualities. There will be implied terms of the partnership which may be inferred from the 1890 Act or from the conduct of the partners to each other.

Many clauses in a written partnership agreement are straightforward and obvious. The agreement must include the names of the partners and title of the partnership. Most GPs conduct their business using their true names. However, if GPs are in partnership and the business name does not reflect the true surnames of all the partners, the 1985 Business Names Act requires the partnership to disclose the true name of each partner and this information would have to be provided on the business correspondence which the partnership normally uses to conduct general medical practice. Discriminatory as it might seem, the effect of the 1985 Act is to require a married woman GP, who conducts her professional medical activities under her maiden name, to abide by these requirements and provide her married name. The partnership agreement should also provide the practice address and the addresses of any branch surgeries where the partnership conducts business. The nature of the business must be defined in order to place a limit upon the actions that each partner can take on behalf of the 'firm'.

The partnership agreement will show the date of the commencement of the partnership and also the date on which the partners have signed the agreement. The recording of these dates might become important if subsequently there is a dispute or simple confusion arising out of the terms of a verbal agreement which varies from the original written agreement.

Many partnerships in the commercial world are of limited duration. In general medical partnership, there is no value in limiting the duration of the partnership, since this reduces the level of security each partner expects. It could lead to a situation where partners anticipate the dissolution of the partnership and compete among themselves instead of working together for the good of the business. As the 1890 Partnership Act states that 'every partnership is dissolved as regards all the partners by the death or bankruptcy of any partner', it is very important that the partnership agreement provides a clause that prevents the partnership from automatically ending with the death of one of the partners. Therefore, a good partnership agreement will include a clause that provides for the duration of the partnership to continue during the joint lives of at least two of the partners who are party to the partnership agreement. The question of how an individual partner may leave the partnership is dealt with below, but it is important to note that a written partnership agreement does not require a specific clause dealing with dissolution. If the partners wish to dissolve the partnership, they can do so at any time by mutual consent.

Obligations of the partners

Each partner would normally be expected to contribute equally to the work of the partnership business. Even if not explicitly stated, there is an implicit obligation placed upon each partner to devote himself fully to the work of the business. Where one or more partners are unable to give as much time as other partners to the work of the business, it is important that the agreement should include provision for this. This also raises the difficult issue of work undertaken outside the partnership. As the assumption is that all the partners are working for the benefit of the partnership, it is usual to make provision for the partnership to give consent to individual partners wishing to undertake other activities, such as clinical assistantships or occupational health sessions. Consent for such work should not be unreasonably withheld.

Regardless of the provisions in the partnership agreement, each partner will have to satisfy the FHSA requirements with regard to minimum commitments for the purposes of their eligibility for BPA. The 1990 contract provides for part-time practitioners who may be three-quarter time or half-time. This is explained fully in Chapter 37.

Partnership and other income

In the same way that each partner is expected to share equally in the work of a business, so each partner may expect to receive an equal share of the profit and to share equally in the capital assets of the business. However, the income which each partner will enjoy derives from the total income of the partnership after expenses have been paid. What then constitutes the income of the partnership? It has been argued that the most appropriate arrangement is that all fees and professional earnings constitute the receipts for partnership income. A partner who is able to retain a certain source of income, particularly when the income is significant, may devote more time to that work and neglect his or her commitment to the partnership. Such behaviour might breach the terms of the partnership agreement whereby a partner gives full attention to the business.

There is also a considerable risk that competition might develop within the partnership as partners compete for certain kinds of income in a locality. This could soon lead to disharmony. In some practices certain receipts may be retained personally by individual partners, notably seniority payments and postgraduate education allowances. Where such arrangements exist, it is vital that they are spelled out within the terms of the partnership agreement, so that each partner is aware of the sources of income that will be treated as partnership receipts and those that will be considered personal to the partner earning them.

Profit-sharing

Having determined what will constitute the income of the partnership, how should the partners share the profits of the business? First, the partnership agreement should identify clearly the expenses that are to be treated as partnership expenses and which will be deducted from the total income before the profit share takes place. There may be variations among practices with regard to what is treated as a partnership expense, and partnerships will be guided by their accountant as to what is most tax advantageous. The share of profits to which each partner is entitled would normally be based on the share of the work undertaken by that partner. The normal expectation is that all partners share equally in the work of the practice and, therefore, all partners share equally in the division of profits. Hitherto, the FHSA has recognized a partnership only when it can be demonstrated that the share of the profits held by any one partner is not less than one-third of the share of the partner who receives the greatest share. For instance, an incoming partner might receive a 10% share of the profits, whereas the other three partners receive 30% each. This fulfils the FHSA requirements. However, the regulations have been amended with effect from 1 April 1990 to take account of three-quarter time and half-time practitioners. This is explained in more detail in Chapter 37.

Most new partners expect to move to parity within a reasonable time; nowadays it is not unusual to achieve parity within three years. The move towards parity is based upon the assumption that the new partner undertakes an equal share of the work in the partnership. It is possible that a partner never achieves parity because he has a limited commitment and is not expected to contribute equally to the work of the practice. Sometimes such doctors are incorrectly termed 'salaried partners'. Such a position does not exist in the regulations and, within the context of a general medical practice partnership, the term is an oxymoron: if one is salaried, one is not a partner. However, the phrase is at times employed as shorthand for a partner with a guaranteed minimum income or fixed sum income, in order to fulfil the FHSA requirement on the one-third rule. Such a partner's income should be described in the partnership agreement as being set at a certain income level or at one-third (or one-quarter or one-fifth—*see* Chapter 37) of the profit share of the partner with the greatest share of profit, whichever is the greater. It is now more acceptable to refer to such doctors as 'fixed share partners'.

Where parity is not reached within a reasonable time, and all partners are contributing equally to the work of the practice, it may be argued that the incoming partner has been the subject of a concealed sale of goodwill.

Capital assets

The 1890 Act provides for partnership and capital shares to be held in the same proportions save where there is an express agreement to the contrary. A sound partnership agreement spells out clearly the obligations placed upon the new partner with regard to buying into the capital of the partnership. An explanation of how one contributes towards the capital of a partnership is given in Chapter 30.

There are two additional points affecting the capital assets of a partnership. First, how does the partnership deal with the capital share of a partner who leaves the partnership? The outgoing partner will want to realize the capital share that has been held in the partnership to date. For the remaining partners it is vital that no ambiguity should exist regarding who owns the capital of the partnership. A partnership agreement will normally provide for the outgoing partner's share of the capital to be purchased by the remaining partners. They in turn would expect to pass this obligation on to the new partner who joins the practice, but this may not be true for every case in which a partnership loses one of its partners.

The second major issue is the valuation of capital assets. Any such valuation should be undertaken by independent qualified valuers. Its basis should be established within the partnership agreement. The valuation must *not* include an element for the sale or purchase of goodwill within the practice. This has been made unlawful under current NHS legislation. Any GP about to enter a partnership, who believes that there may be an element of goodwill in the price asked for his capital share, is advised to seek the assistance of the Medical Practices Committee, which is able to certify that a sale of goodwill is not involved in a particular transaction. If a partner contributes equally to the work of the business but never achieves parity, such a disproportionate share of profits may be interpreted as a concealed sale of goodwill, which is treated in the same way as the inclusion of an element of goodwill in the valuation of capital assets within a practice.

Practice premises are discussed in detail in Chapters 27 and 28. A sound partnership agreement should include a clause on the practice premises and take account of lease arrangements, rental agreements, and so on.

Decision-making

The decision-making process in the partnership requires considerable attention in the partnership agreement. Often, it is a source of friction within the partnership, arising from a failure to detail the various obligations placed upon the partnership when making decisions. If there is no clear statement regarding decision-making within the partnership, then the decision-making process is subject to the provisions of the 1890 Partnership Act. This would mean that: (i) no partner may be introduced as a partner without the consent of all existing partners, and (ii) normal business matters will be decided by a majority vote of the partners. The partnership agreement should make clear which decisions require the unanimous consent of all partners. In addition to the admission of a new partner, it is advisable to make the dismissal of any practice staff a matter for unanimous decision. In the event of any subsequent application to an industrial tribunal by a former member of staff who believes he has been unfairly dismissed, the partnership will be liable. The question of majority decision-making on everyday matters can sometimes present problems. In large partnerships of, say, eight principals, a majority decision might still have three partners in disagreement. It may therefore be thought appropriate to identify certain kinds of decisions which would require a two-thirds majority to take effect.

Holiday, study and sickness leave

A doctor employed within the NHS has annual leave, sick leave payments and arrangements for maternity leave clearly laid down. In general medical partnership, it is up to the partnership to decide on these matters. The partnership agreement should provide for all partners to enjoy equal amounts of annual leave which the partnership should decide, although the new regulations place an upper limit of six weeks' annual leave for a principal on the FHSA list. The partnership may also decide whether there should be a limit on the amount of annual leave to be taken at any one time and may consider the advisability of having arrangements for annual leave that limit the number of partners absent at any one time. The same consideration should apply to the granting of study leave within the partnership, particularly where prolonged study leave, as defined in paragraph 50.1 – 50.17 of the SFA, is contemplated.

Study leave and annual leave can be planned in advance. Absence arising from sick leave will rarely by anticipated. It is important that the partnership agreement includes arrangements to cover for sickness absences within the partnership. Although there is no single arrangement that can be recommended, it is normal practice for the partner absent on sick leave to pay the costs of locum cover where the sickness absence exceeds, for example, a period of two weeks. The advantage of such a formula is that normally the individual partners will pay lower premiums on their personal sickness insurance policies. The sick leave clause should also take account of the arrangements described in the SFA with regard to payment for locum cover during the sickness of a partner where the criteria described (paragraph 48.1 – 48.27) in the SFA are met.

Maternity leave

Maternity leave provisions are a major consideration in partnership at a time when four out of 10 doctors entering general practice are women. The statutory provision for maternity leave does not apply to a principal in general practice, who is not an employee. Neither is the principal in general practice eligible for the extensive range of maternity leave provisions to which female staff in the NHS are entitled. Instead, it is the responsibility of the partnership to determine the arrangements which it wishes to apply where a female partner requires leave arising from her pregnancy.

Where a sickness or maternity allowance is received from the FHSA, the disposal of it should follow the payment of the locum fees for the comparable period.

It is to be expected that a female partner would want to clarify possible arrangements arising from her pregnancy. There are a variety of options that partnerships may apply in these circumstances. One note of caution has to be sounded. The 1986 Sex Discrimination Act makes unlawful the treatment

of a female who is pregnant in a way that is less favourable than the treatment of the incapacity of a male arising from a condition peculiar to men.
When framing the provisions for maternity leave, partnerships should take
account of the provisions to be found in paragraphs 49.1 – 49.12 of the SFA.
In summary, a practice may claim for up to 13 weeks' locum cover for a
female partner absent as a result of pregnancy. The broad conditions are
similar to those for payment made during sickness; however, the female
partner absent during her confinement does not have to fulfil the criteria
regarding the remaining average list size. Certain adjustments are also made
for three-quarter and half-time practitioners.

Maternity leave clauses should provide for an appropriate continuing
income for the absent female partner and appropriate locum cover for the
work of the partnership. One simple solution is to permit the female partner
to continue to receive her share of the profits, whilst being responsible for the
payment of a locum during her period of absence. The arrangements should
also take account of the need for ante-natal care, a minimum period of leave
afforded to the absent female partner, and a limit placed upon the total
period of the absence which the woman partner may take. Where the woman
partner is involved in a job-share (*see* Chapter 37), account should be taken
of this in the maternity leave arrangements. If she is a part-time practitioner
as defined in the regulations, this does not affect her right to be treated in the
same way as a whole-time practitioner for the purposes of maternity leave
arrangements.

Leaving the partnership

A good partnership agreement provides security for all the partners and for
the partnership as a whole. However, this does not mean that an individual
doctor should be tied throughout his working life to a particular partnership.
Similarly GPs would not wish to remain in partnership with somebody
whose behaviour and actions are unacceptable. The provision for partners
to retire voluntarily is straightforward. The expulsion of an unsuitable
partner can be problematic. The most important aspect of a voluntary
retirement clause is to ensure that the outgoing partner gives sufficient notice
to the partnership. The minimum notice should be three months since the
FHSA requires this if the outgoing partner intends to resign from the FHSA
list. The recruitment and replacement timetable can extend beyond three
months and it is not unusual to find that a departing partner is required to
give six months' notice. Obviously this period of notice can be varied by
mutual agreement within the partnership.

Expulsion of a partner is an unpleasant problem for any partnership. The 1890 Act requires an express agreement within the partnership to permit the majority of partners to expel a partner. However, the reasons for an expulsion must be sound and demonstrably justify the act of expulsion. Hence expulsion clauses normally list circumstances that may include:

- removal from the FHSA list
- suspension or erasure from the GMC register
- grossly immoral conduct
- habitual insobriety
- bankruptcy
- neglect of the practice
- breaches of medical ethics
- compulsory detention under the Mental Health Act 1983
- lengthy incapacity leave from work.

Whilst matters such as erasure from the GMC register or removal from the FHSA list are clear-cut, judgements made with regard to the neglect of the practice or lengthy incapacity leave from work can be very difficult. It is therefore recommended that any partner served with an expulsion order by the remaining partners should have the opportunity to take the matter to arbitration as provided for elsewhere in the partnership agreement.

A partner may also be required to leave the partnership upon reaching a pre-determined retirement age established by the partnership agreement. However, compulsory retirement ages are rarely found in partnership agreements and it may be that the new retirement rules incorporated into the revised regulations will be seen as sufficient for the purposes of compulsory retirement.

Whether a partner leaves voluntarily or is expelled, there arises the question of placing a restraint on the outgoing partner. Such a restraint is designed to protect the goodwill of the partnership since, although the goodwill cannot be sold or purchased, there is no prohibition on its protection. This restraint clause is commonly known as a restrictive covenant. There has been considerable controversy over the years regarding the reliance that can be placed on restrictive covenants. Some GPs feel that these are unenforceable. However, whilst the courts have judged how reasonable a restrictive covenant is, there is no doubt that a reasonable restraint clause will be upheld. Almost 40 years ago, a restraint clause that prohibited the outgoing GP from practising for a 21-year period within a 10-mile radius of the main surgery, was upheld by the courts. It is unimaginable that such a clause would be upheld nowadays. However, clauses that restrain the outgoing partner from practising as a general medical practitioner for, say, one year within a defined geographical area around the main surgery, are likely to be upheld in the courts. The precise geographical area will vary, since in a very rural practice with a scattered population, a radius of three or four miles might be reasonable, whereas that same radius in an inner city practice might be considered unnecessarily restrictive. Although restraint clauses are subject to the test of reasonableness, it is also likely in the future that they will be judged against the question of restricting competition for new business, and whether that attempt to prevent competition goes beyond the legitimate attempt by the existing business to protect its interests.

General medical practice is not immune from litigation by aggrieved patients or relatives. Consequently it is in the interest of a partnership that the agreement requires each partner to maintain membership of a defence body. Some partnership agreements require the partners to maintain their membership for a specified number of years after leaving the partnership. This is not necessary since defence bodies' subscriptions cover the GP during the period of that subscription and if membership subsequently ceases following retirement, for example, any claim relating to the period of the subscription will be honoured by the defence body.

Summary and sources of advice

No written partnership agreement can be a guarantee of harmony within the partnership. Consequently a sound partnership agreement will include an arbitration clause. This will permit serious disputes within the partnership to be referred to an independent arbitrator nominated by the Secretary of the BMA. Where disputes of a minor kind arise, the partners can seek the advice of their LMC or BMA local office.

Partnership is not a series of agreements written down and accepted by all the partners. Partnership is a relationship that exists between the GPs who come together to form a partnership; it is a legal relationship and, as such, other people and institutions will have certain expectations of the partnership as a whole. For the partnership to work, all the partners must be committed to it and devote themselves to its development and success. The test of a sound partnership is that it should provide harmony, security, equity, and the basis of mutual trust and confidence. The successful partnership is probably the one that is least likely to need to refer to a written partnership agreement. However, no partnership can afford the risk of not having a sound written partnership agreement to provide a clear under-standing of the duties and obligatons of each partner.

When entering into partnership, GPs should take expert advice. This may come from the practice solicitor, although a new partner may wish to obtain advice from his own solicitor before committing himself to the terms of the partnership agreement. Partnership advice is readily available from the LMC and from the BMA's industrial relations officers. Advice is available throughout the whole process of partnership, from the first decision to draw up a partnership agreement to offering advice and assistance with disputes including serious differences which may arise within the partnership. Such advice is vital to the GP trainee who has been accustomed to the world of employment and is entering partnership as an independent contractor for the first time. It is vitally important for that GP to understand the implications of partnership, the obligations it places upon him and the fact that in partnership a group of GPs are working together for their mutual benefit; they are not working alone and they are not working against each other. Consequently, when a dispute arises within a partnership it should be possible for the partnership as a whole to seek advice in order to resolve that dispute. The BMA's industrial relations officers are always available to offer that help and can obtain further expert advice from the Association's specialist departments. There is nothing to be gained from adopting en-trenched positions and treating partners as 'the enemy'. There is much to be gained in seeking expert advice and a sympathetic ear at the first hint of serious difficulty.

23 The New Partner

As has been discussed in Chapter 21, the vast majority of GPs in this country practise as members of groups or, more commonly, partnerships, which usually involve the pooling of all earnings and the division of profits between the partners on a prescribed—normally fractional—basis. Indeed, the division of profits by this means is the main characteristic of the true partnership.

In some circumstances (*see* page 165), practice profits are shared according to a different scale to those arising from surgery ownership. An example of such an arrangement in a typical six-doctor partnership is set out below.

	Surgery income %	Practice profits %
Dr A	25	18
Dr B	25	18
Dr C	25	18
Dr D	25	18
Dr E	–	15
Dr F	–	13
	100	100

In this particular example, the four senior partners only own the surgery and retain the net income arising from that ownership. Drs E and F are younger partners working towards parity.

Medical partnerships by their nature are dynamic. The ages of the partners are likely to be progressive, so that a partner may retire every few years and there is consequently a regular inflow of new partners. In addition, partners may leave through disagreements or early retirement, or a partner may die in service. These variables generate a pattern of fairly regular partnership changes.

In contrast to other professions, where a person would have to be known well, possibly for many years, before being offered a partnership, the nature of general practice, with its system of practice allowances and payments only to principals, means that young doctors join as partners from their date of appointment. As a result, some partnerships do not hold together, and the new partner may leave at the end of his probationary period. If the level of list sizes calls for another doctor, however, the practice is penalized by the denial of a practice allowance, if he is not a partner at once. The introduction of a new partner is also likely to result in a substantial saving in locum fees and deputizing costs, which will increase the profit available for distribution between the partners.

Figure 23.1 shows how the introduction of an additional partner into a practice affects its financial organization and profit-sharing ratios. The size of the partnership increases from four to five partners, and the new partner commences on an annual income of £20 000, which after a six-month pro-bationary period will be converted to a percentage share of 10.8%, rising in equal steps to parity over three years. Some practices offer an incoming partner parity after only six months, but this is the exception rather than the rule.

Another decision which must be taken at the outset is whether the partners are to retain their own seniority and postgraduate education allowances. Again, this is at the discretion of the partners, although most practices adopt the policy of paying such awards to the partners in whose names they are paid, rather than pooling them with partnership profits for division. Whatever policy is adopted, it should be the same for all partners; it should be clearly laid down in the partnership deed and reflected as such in the partnership accounts (*see* page 102).

'Salaried' and 'fixed-share' partners

It is still relatively common for GPs to be paid their share of the profits on a 'fixed-share' rather than a fractional or equity basis. Doctors to whom this normally applies are new partners still in their probationary period, part-time (usually women) doctors and senior doctors who have taken a 24-hour retirement. These doctors are sometimes referred to as 'salaried partners', but this term has connotations of employment which are best avoided for taxation and other reasons.

The criterion in medical practice, that determines whether or not a doctor is a partner, is eligibility for the BPA. This is paid only to principals in general practice and a doctor who is engaged on such a basis and has fulfilled all the requirements is a partner, regardless of how he is remunerated.

Such a partner should therefore, after an initial probationary period, play a full part in the management of the practice. Administrative or other duties should be delegated to him; his name should appear on the practice notepaper; he should attend partnership meetings; he should be a signatory

Drs Bass, Truman and Partners

Profits per accounts to 31 March 1993
Add: Projected increase: 1993/94 (2%)

	Total earnings
	£
Profits per accounts to 31 March 1993	175 000
Add: Projected increase: 1993/94 (2%)	3500
	178 500
	180 000

	Probationary period From 1 Apr 1993		First year (1) From 1 Oct 1993		Second year From 1 Oct 1994		Third year From 1 Oct 1995		Fourth year From 1 Oct 1996	
	%	£	%	£ (2)	%	£ (2)	%	£ (2)	%	£
Dr Bass	25	40 000	22.3	41 500	21.55	41 807	20.8	42 432	20	42 840
Dr Truman	25	40 000	22.3	41 500	21.55	41 807	20.8	42 432	20	42 840
Dr Young	25	40 000	22.3	41 500	21.55	41 807	20.8	42 432	20	42 840
Dr Watney	25	40 000	22.3	41 500	21.55	41 807	20.8	42 432	20	42 840
New partner	–	20 000	10.8	20 000	13.80	26 772	16.8	34 272	20	42 840
	100	180 000	100.0	186 000	100.00	194 000	100.0	204 000	100	214 200

(1) Assuming an annual increase of profits at 5% per annum.
(2) Figures have been rounded where necessary.

Figure 23.1 Future shares of profit on the introduction of a new partner from 1 April 1993 at an initial remuneration of £20 000, rising to parity over three years

to the partnership bank account, and generally be treated as an equal by his colleagues.

In order also to fulfil the rules laid down by the NHS, no partner should be paid less than one-third of the income of the highest paid partner and all should work at least 26 hours in the practice (except part-time partners: *see* Chapter 37). As indicated above, the NHS requires that all partners share in the management of the practice.

The introduction of capital

A GP joining a practice is likely to be required to contribute to the capital of the practice. How much that will be depends upon the nature of the partnership, eg whether it is a property owning partnership, a dispensing practice or a highly capitalized business with a lot of office and medical equipment.

The new partner should also ensure that he is registered for National Insurance purposes (*see* Chapter 44). He should take steps immediately to ensure that HM Inspector of Taxes is advised of his position so that he is charged his proper share of the partnership tax assessment (*see* Chapter 39). He is likely also to be invited to sign a continuation election.

Before appointment, the prospective partner should ask to see the partnership accounts for the immediate past accounting period, and there is no reason why these should be withheld from him. He should also ask to see a copy of the partnership deed.

24 Financing a New Doctor

Most general practices, at some time, face the problem of how to cater for expansion in the practice. Such expansion can arise for a number of reasons: the practice may be in an expanding area with a great deal of new building taking place; it may have attracted patients from other practices by offering better facilities; or the introduction of new and younger partners may have encouraged patients to join who may not otherwise have done so. Some practices, for instance, have found that their popularity is increased by the introduction of a female partner.

If a partner leaves the practice, causing a drop in the number of partners, the remaining doctors must decide whether they need to recruit a new partner. Some practices have reasoned that if, for example, six partners can cater for 12 000 patients at an average of 2000 each, five partners should not have too much trouble in taking on 400 extra patients each. Some practices have indeed chosen to take that course. These tend to be practices made up of younger partners who do not object to taking on an additional workload. This has been encouraged by the 1990 GP contract, which initiated a reduction in the BPA, from just under £13 000 (or more if a vocational training allowance was added) in 1989/90, to £6000 in the first year of the new contract.

Nevertheless, some partnerships find they cannot continue with their present number of doctors, and seek to recruit an additional person to share the workload. There are a number of ways in which this can be done, and the financial consequences of all options should be considered.

Figure 24.1 compares three options for a four-doctor practice which needs help to cope with its expanding workload. In the year 1992/93, the practice earned a total of £200 000, an average of £50 000 each. For the purpose of these calculations, it is assumed that such items as seniority, PGEA and cost rent allowances are shared in other ratios, and they have been excluded from the calculation. The practice has a total of 10 800 patients, or 2700 per partner. The eldest partner, at 45 years, still has family commitments; therefore the partnership is reluctant to burden itself with the potential dilution of its profits by taking on an additional partner. It has considered recruiting a locum or an assistant doctor and has estimated the cost of either at £20 000 per annum. It has also considered recruiting an additional partner.

The practice has already been paying out £10 000 per annum to part-time locums, who have worked when required during periods of holidays and sickness. The recruitment of an additional doctor would dispense with this cost.

Locum fees

The partners have been advised that if they appoint a locum, and pay him a regular salary, then they will be required to pay the employer's share of his Class 1 National Insurance contributions. They would prefer not to do this, and to avoid it must make sure that the locums they employ are assessable to Schedule D tax on their earnings, ie they must be effectively self-employed. The cost to the partners of this arrangement would be £20 000, but from this would be deducted the £10 000 presently paid to part-time locums.

A regular locum may not be accepted by the FHSA as an assistant and would therefore be unable to attract an assistant's allowance.

An assistant

An assistant is an employee of the practice; he or she will be in an employer – employee relationship to the practice, which will be responsible for deducting PAYE tax from the salary and for the employer's share of the Class 1 NIC. At a salary of £20 000 this would represent an additional cost of 10.4% or £2080. The practice would, however, subject to agreement of the FHSA, be able to attract the assistant's allowance for a non-designated area of £5790 for 1993/94.

A new partner

The introduction of a new partner is in many ways the most satisfactory solution. The practice will, in theory, save the locum fees previously paid, but will attract another BPA (presently £6624) without any additional costs except the payment to the new partner of his share in the profits. However, the desirability of this option will depend on the new partner's share of the profits and progression to parity. In the example given, it is assumed that he will be recruited at an initial share of 10%, rising to parity over three years by two equal and intermediate steps before achieving parity at 20% of the profits.

Four full-time GPs; average profits £50 000, after paying locum fees of £10 000;
10 800 patients

	Present position (1992/93) £	New position (1993/94) Locum £	Assistant £	Partner £
Partnership profit	200 000	200 000	200 000	200 000
Add: Inflation @ 7%	–	8000	8000	8000
Basic Practice Allowance	–	–	–	6624
Assistant's allowance	–	–	5790	–
Saving in locum fees (part-time)	–	10 000	10 000	10 000
	200 000	218 000	223 790	230 624
Less: Locum fees	–	20 000	–	–
Assistant's salary	–	–	20 000	–
Class 1 NIC (10.4%)	–	–	2080	–
	200 000	198 000	201 710	224 624
Profit shares: 4 partners each:				
1992/93	50 000			
1993/94		49 500	50 428	
New partner @ 10%				22 462 (1)
4 partners (each)				50 540

(1) This share will increase by stages (probably over 3 years) until the new partner achieves
parity.

Figure 24.1   Comparative costs for a four-doctor practice taking on a locum, assistant or
fifth partner

Comparison of results

It may be seen from the calculation in Figure 24.1 that, using the locum
route, the partners will each receive a share of the profits of £49 500, which
represents a slight fall from their previous year's income. This may be
thought worthwhile, bearing in mind the saving in the workload entailed.

The recruitment of an assistant, however, will attract a potential income
of £50 428 each, or an increase of about 1%.

The recruitment of a partner will result in an almost indentical rate of
increase, but there are other advantages which accrue. The partners would
assure the succession of the practice and, if there is a surgery ownership
situation, they may be able to pass on a share of this to the incoming partner
in due course. Unless there is likely to be a fall in the list sizes, which seems
unlikely, the partners will have a continuing average of 2160 patients

(somewhat above the national average). The permanence of a new partner is also a guarantee of stability. However, the new partner's share of the profits will rise fairly sharply over a three-year period, and this could reduce the shares of the other partners in real terms unless they are able to attract new sources of income.

The tax advantages of new partner recruitment are discussed below.

Taxation

A partnership increasing its size is in a highly advantageous situation for tax purposes. As the assessment is based on the profits of the preceding year, five partners may be assessed on profits earned by four. In our example, therefore, and discounting all other variables, the five-doctor practice will, in the year 1993–4, pay tax on profits of £200 000, which were earned by four partners in the previous year. At such a time, the partnership will be earning an overall net income that is 11% higher than that of the previous year. This potential tax advantage is significant and should not be discounted.

The new partner himself will derive a substantial taxation benefit from being assessed to tax under Schedule D, rather than Schedule E (PAYE), which would apply if he were an assistant.

The figures in Figure 24.1 are not necessarily representative, but are deployed solely to illustrate the above points, and practices should adapt them to their own needs. It is advisable to consult the practice accountant, as he or she will be in a position to supply accurate figures.

25 Joining a Practice

THE majority of those entering a general practice partnership for the first time will be doing so shortly after completing a general practice vocational training scheme. During training, a practitioner may form an idea of what his ideal practice will be. When the search begins for an ideal practice, it is helpful if the practitioner concerned has decided upon a range of features that are considered vital, some features that may be desirable, and those elements which, if necessary, may be amended in the light of the opportunities that present themselves.

Choosing a practice

The location of a practice will determine to a significant extent the life-styles of the GP and the population served. The spectrum ranges from rural dispensing practices, through semi-rural and suburban practices, to inner city practices serving areas of high social deprivation. The prospective principal must decide what his or her aptitudes and skills are best suited for. The rural practice will almost certainly offer a pleasant environment, perhaps the possibility of participating in the work of a cottage hospital, and the opportunity to become part of the social life of the area. Balanced against this could be the disadvantages of professional isolation, less choice of staff to assist in the running of the practice, and reduced opportunity for maintaining close contact with large district general hospitals.

The practitioner seeking an urban practice may be looking for the challenge of serving a population subject to a range of social disadvantages, perhaps the opportunity to become involved in the academic activities of university departments and teaching hospitals, and the greater contact with the profession generally offered by the high GP population in urban areas.

Geographical location may also determine the level of competition for each vacancy. Competition for vacancies in general practice is keen and the competition for particularly attractive vacancies may appear daunting. A practitioner is fortunate if he obtains the first vacancy for which he applies. It is usual for a prospective principal to make a series of applications before being successful. During a period of unsuccessful applications, it is tempting to make compromises over the 'ideal' practice. It is important that the practitioner judges in advance those features over which a compromise is possible, and those where he is not prepared to compromise.

How can suitable vacancies be identified? First impressions will be gained from information available from course organizers, FHSAs or an advertisement. Similarly, a written application will be the first impression that a partnership gains of a candidate. How then should an application for a vacancy in general practice be submitted? As dozens of applications may be submitted, it is important to provide a letter of application and curriculum vitae that tell a practice something about the candidate, and which command its interest.

The curriculum vitae

Studies undertaken by personnel professionals indicate that the average time spent looking at each job application is less than one minute. In that time a judgement is made regarding whether the applicant is suitable for the job being advertised. A curriculum vitae must contain information about personal details and qualifications and experience in medicine.

Personal details should include the following.

- Name and address, nationality, date of birth and age.
- Marital status.
- Possession of current driving licence.
- State of health.
- Professional qualifications and medical experience, including period of attendance at university and medical school with details of any distinctions or prizes obtained.
- Date of full registration with the GMC.
- A list of all medical appointments held, starting with the most recent and listing them in reverse chronological order, including any special service such as military or VSO.
- Details of current employment, and availability to enter general practice.
- Any special experience.
- Membership or Fellowship of Royal Colleges or Faculties.
- Other postgraduate qualifications.
- Details of research or published articles, including special interests pursued while undertaking hospital jobs or general practice vocational training.
- Interests outside medicine, particularly the gaining of any distinction, in sport, for example.
- The names, addresses and telephone numbers of referees, who must always include the candidate's trainer and course organizer.

A curriculum vitae should be professionally typed and clearly set out, with appropriate margins or spacings left for those who shortlist and interview to make comments and notes. The letter accompanying the curriculum vitae should be handwritten, legible, and provide a personal perspective on the reasons for the application, including the candidate's particular interest in the practice vacancy and the location of the practice.

An application may result in one or more interviews at the practice. A good practice will provide a practice profile in advance to give you basic information that can be added to when attending the practice for interview. It is not unusual for an applicant to be subjected to an initial interview which provides the practice with the opportunity to draw up a short-list for final selection.

Questions to ask

What questions should a doctor ask when invited to an interview? Of paramount importance is information regarding the partners with whom, if successful, the doctor may be working for the rest of his professional life. The candidate should find out how many there are, their ages, how the partnership vacancy arose, how the partnership conducts its management of the practice, and what sort of new partner they are seeking.

An immediate impression of the premises will be gained on the first visit. If it is a health centre, the doctor should ascertain the lease arrangements with the health authority. If the property is owned by the partnership, questions will be needed about the incoming partner's obligations with regard to the financing of the premises and the purchase of the capital share of those premises. The doctor should satisfy himself that the premises, furnishings and equipment within the practice appear in good condition, that there are facilities for the staff and that the practice as a whole is equipped to deal with its list of patients. He should also enquire about any particular difficulties with the premises, such as a lack of parking space for the partners.

It is important to learn about the practice staff: how many staff are employed by the practice and do the staff include a practice nurse or other health professionals? Is there a practice administrator or manager, and does the practice issue formal written contracts and job descriptions for its staff? Are there staff who are attached to the practice, for example a health visitor or a social worker? What is the usual method of communicating with staff members? Does any one partner have a particular responsibility for staff and personnel matters? The candidate will note how the staff treated him when he first arrived at the practice.

Questions regarding financial matters are dealt with in detail elsewhere. A doctor will wish to be satisfied that the financial affairs of the practice are in good order and accordingly will require some idea about the accounts within the practice, the main sources of income of the practice, and any major financial obligations which the practice is taking on or may take on in the near future.

An applicant for a vacancy should find out about the partnership arrangements: it is important to establish whether there is a written partnership agreement and what it states about the major issues discussed in Chapter 22.

No practice operates in total isolation and it is therefore important to establish the relationships the practice has with the FHSA, the LMC, local hospitals and their consultants, other practices, and the social services department of the local authority. If the area is unfamiliar, it is important to find out about the local housing market, ease of travel, schooling, banks and shopping facilities.

The interview

Generally, the most difficult hurdle in the process of joining a new practice is the interview. An invitation to interview indicates that an applicant has passed the first hurdle and that the written application has succeeded in 'selling' that doctor. At the interview, the process of selling oneself continues, but it is equally important that the interview creates a two-way process by which the partners can judge the applicant and the applicant can reflect on whether he wishes to join that partnership. A good interview will be a relaxed and friendly affair, but sufficiently businesslike to ensure that candidates can be properly assessed and interviewers judged. First impressions count. The candidate who is dressed for the occasion and is positive and direct in manner, will impress at the outset. Preparation is also vital and, where the applicant has been sent material in advance, it should be obvious whether the material has been read and understood. It is particularly important that the candidate should be ready to answer questions where the application reveals an earlier interest or commitment to a career in hospital medicine, or where there appear to be unexplained gaps in the employment chronology. Candidates will always be asked if they have any questions themselves and it is common sense to prepare two or three questions in advance. This should not inhibit asking questions during the course of the interview, provided that this does not mean that the interviewing panel are unable to get through all the questions they have planned to ask.

Throughout the interview, the main question that the interviewers and the applicant will have at the back of their minds is 'Can I get on with this person?'. The answer to that question will arise from the manner and conduct at the interview, from the way in which the applicants 'come over', how open they are, how truthful they are, and how committed they appear to the vacancy on offer. Where part of the interviewing process involves the applicant's spouse, it is important to ensure that the applicant and spouse do not put across conflicting messages to the partnership. There is no point in a doctor applying for a post emphasizing the advantage placed upon the value of life in a rural practice if the spouse has interests and commitments which can be fulfilled only in an urban environment.

If successful, the new partner will be subject to a probationary period, commonly called a period of mutual assessment. This may last for between three and 12 months, and provides for a period in which neither side to a new agreement is making a final commitment. The new partner has a chance to measure his expectations of the practice against the reality, and the partnership taking in a new doctor will be able to judge whether the interviewing process has successfully identified the correct candidate for the post. Although it is rare for the period of mutual assessment not to lead to continuing partnership with the new partner, it provides an important safeguard for all concerned and can avoid the trauma and difficulty associated with the departure of a partner under the arrangements described in Chapter 22.

26 Calculating the Partners' Drawings

IN all partnerships there must be a system of withdrawing funds from the practice account by the partners, so that income can be passed to their own accounts for personal use. Doctors, like all other sections of the community, have their personal living expenses to finance and there must be a regular and controlled means of transferring funds to them.

For employees, such as hospital doctors, GP trainees and consultants, this is not a problem. Their salaries will normally be paid to them at the end of each month, having undergone all necessary deductions. GPs, however, are not employees; as we have seen, they are self-employed individuals and, as partners, they have a responsibility to each other. One of these is to ensure that funds passed to them from time to time are in keeping both with their profit-sharing ratios and all other known factors.

Unfortunately, incorrect terminology is often used; it is highly misleading when doctors refer to the monthly amounts paid to them as their 'salary'. This is not the case and the fact cannot be emphasized too strongly. The word 'salary' has all manner of unfortunate connotations in this context, not least being the manner in which the income is taxed, and it is better to avoid the term if at all possible.

It is no exaggeration to say that the periodic calculation of partnership drawings is one of the financial procedures which regularly causes most difficulties to GPs in partnership. Many doctors feel that knowledge of their incomes is of such a confidential nature that it cannot be delegated to a member of their staff. These calculations are therefore, in many cases, done by one of the partners themselves. Fortunately, attitudes are changing and, in an increasing number of cases, such drawings calculations are done by a responsible practice manager.

Rather different problems concern the single-handed practitioner. He has no partners to worry about and the money he earns is his own, subject of course to making prudent provisions for income tax and other matters. He may, however, be well advised to pass all his professional transactions through a separate practice bank account and to transfer monthly such sums as can reasonably be set aside into his private bank account for his own use.

Drawings calculations should be done correctly, if partners are to avoid feeling they are receiving more or less than their proper entitlement, and in order to avoid disparities in their current accounts at the end of each financial year.

Whether drawings have been properly calculated or not will become evident when the annual partnership accounts are prepared; any differences between the current accounts of the partners will then become apparent. Steps should be taken to see that such errors do not recur and that the balances are adjusted by subsequent and 'one-off' adjustments to drawings.

There are probably as many different systems of drawings by partners as there are fingers on one's hands. Whatever system is used, it is essential that it is operated properly. The simplest system would apply in a two-man partnership sharing profits equally, so that both doctors could withdraw identical amounts. In practice, that is likely to be the exception rather than the rule. In virtually all cases, complex adjustments will be made for differing rates of seniority awards; superannuation payments; added years contributions; loan interest charges; national insurance; repayments of leave advance, and other items.

The system which is perhaps most widely used in partnerships is the 'month-end' or 'quarter-end' system, under which partners are paid out at the end of each month, and adjustments made quarterly to take into consideration the factors mentioned above. Whilst it is acceptable that payments at the end of the two intermediate months may be made in partnership ratios, the full measure of adjustments must be made at the end of the quarter. This is illustrated by the example shown in Figure 26.1. This shows a four-doctor partnership, Drs A, B, C and D, the three senior partners having a share of 28% and a new partner, Dr D, with a share of 16%. Drs A and B are both paying for added years (A); all the partners are paying leave advances (B); whilst Dr D has a loan from the GP Finance Corporation (C). Drs A, B, C and D have seniority awards at varying rates (D). The figures shown are for illustration purposes only and it should not be assumed that these will apply to partnerships in practice.

In computing the total amount to be distributed, it is normal to find the balance available on the partnership bank account (F), either by reference to the bank statements at the end of the quarter or, more preferably and where adequate and accurate records are kept, by referring to the balance in hand as shown in the practice cash book. There should be retained from the amount the estimated expenditure to run the practice during the succeeding months (G), and the balance will then be available for distribution (H).

It should be remembered that, at the same time as this distribution is made, certain deductions have been made from the quarterly FHSA remuneration and, similarly, certain additions will have been included (*see* Box 26.1). It is necessary to reverse these entries before arriving at the total allocation for the quarter and then to allocate the proper amounts to each of the four partners.

Box 26.1: Details of likely items to be adjusted on periodic drawings calculations

Income
- Seniority awards.
- Postgraduate education allowance.
- Notional rent allowance (where to be distributed in different ratios to partnership shares).

Outgoings
- Superannuation contributions: standard.
- Added years and unreduced lump sum.
- National Insurance contributions.
- Repayment of leave advances.
- GPFC (or other loan repayments and interest).
- Transfers to income tax reserve.

It may also be that certain of the partners do not own the surgery premises and they will not be entitled to share in any notional rent allowances in respect of the building. A detailed examination of the quarterly FHSA statement should be made, in order to ensure that all items of this nature are taken into account. Care should also be taken to see that all the income to be distributed has been earned during a period when current profit-sharing ratios were in operation. In many cases, NHS income is paid substantially in arrears. It should ideally be allocated to the period in which it was actually earned and, where such items of income have been received during one quarter, these should be taken out of the normal quarterly calculation and divided separately, in appropriate ratios.

Equalized drawings systems

Many partnerships are now becoming aware of systems of equalized drawings, under which a full year's net income is estimated and divided into equal amounts for distribution to the partners. Provided that all proper adjustments have been made, this regular monthly withdrawal can be paid to the partners' personal bank accounts by standing order.

This system allows a partner to estimate his regular monthly income, for the purpose of his personal family budget, and also avoids the constant calculation and issue of monthly cheques. The system is illustrated in Figure 26.2, for a four-doctor partnership with varying rates of superannuation,

Drs A, B, C and D	Total £	Dr A 28%	Dr B 28%	Dr C 28%	Dr D 16%
Balance in partnership bank account (F)	13 000				
Less:					
retain on hand (G)	4500				
For distribution (H)	8500				
Add deductions:					
Superannuation	540				
Added years (A)	120				
Leave advance (B)	1200				
GPFC loan (C)	125				
Monthly on account	10 000 11 985				
	20 485				
Less additional income:					
Seniority (D)	2800				
For allocation (in partnership ratios)	17 685	4952	4952	4952	2829
Add:					
Seniority (D)	2800	1000	1000	400	400
	20 485	− 5952	− 5952	− 5352	3229
Less:					
Superannuation	540	150	150	150	90
Added years (A)	120	75	45		300
Leave advance (B)	1200	300	300	300	125
GPFC loan (C)	125 1985	− 525	495	450	515
	18 500	5427	5457	4902	2714
Less: paid monthly on account	10 000	2800	2800	2800	1600
Net withdrawals	8500	2627	2657	2102	1114

Figure 26.1   Calculation of quarterly drawings, October 1993

seniority, added years and other items. This calculation is normally made on a tax year basis, so that a reserve (*see* page 162) can be made for the annual partnership income tax liability.

The detailed preparation of such an equalized drawings system will normally be done by the partnership accountant, who should have the required detailed information available to him, and who will be in a position to calculate the tax reserve to be operated during any given period.

	Total	Dr A (28%)	Dr B (28%)	Dr C (24%)	Dr D (20%)
		£	£	£	£
Estimated partnership profits for year	90 000	25 200	25 200	21 600	18 000
Seniority awards	7400	3900	2000	–	1500
Total income (est) (1)	97 400	29 100	27 200	21 600	19 500
Deductions					
Superannuation (est)	5600	1600	1500	1300	1200
Added years	1300	800	300	200	–
Outside appts (est)	100	–	20	80	–
National insurance (est)					
Class I (appointments)	100	–	–	100	–
Class II (stamps)	960	240	240	240	240
Repayment of leave advance	4824	1206	1206	1206	1206
Repayment of loans (GPFC)	1300	–	–	500	800
	14 184	3846	3266	3626	3446
Income tax reserve transfers	18 000	6500	5500	4000	2000
Total outgoings (2)	32 184	10 346	8766	7626	5446
Net (1–2)	65 216	18 754	18 434	13 974	14 054
Monthly	5434	1563	1536	1164	1171
(rounded down)	5415	1560	1530	1160	1165

Figure 26.2 Calculation of equalized drawings for the year to June 1994

The use of income tax reserve accounts

We have had a look at the manner in which drawings calculations are made and that these must take into account the practice's tax liabilities. Tax is normally payable in two instalments on 1 January and 1 July. Many practices, for reasons of cash flow benefit and security, prefer to set regular amounts aside in a separate deposit or building society account, from which these payments might be made as and when they fall due. Systems of this nature have two main advantages.

1 They avoid the drawing of large cheques by individual partners twice a year, often with fairly traumatic effects on the individual's own finances.
2 They avoid the possibility of a retiring partner leaving a tax liability behind him, which may fall on the continuing partners.

The timescale for the operation of such a reserve is important and to a great degree depends on the estimates of future liabilities being received as early as possible within each separate tax year.

Under the normal preceding year basis of assessment, a practice with a year-end on, say 30 June, will find that the profits earned in the year ending on that date will be assessable in the following tax year. In the case of a practice making up its accounts to 30 June 1993, the tax assessment based on those profits would be for the tax year 1994/95. It would normally be possible for an accountant to make a reasonable estimate of the tax payable before the start of the actual year of assessment. With a 31 March year-end, however, it may be May or June before even a preliminary estimate can be prepared.

The reserve should be held physically separate from the main partnership funds, either in a building society or bank deposit account, and the periodic interest divided between the partners in proportion to their shares of the balance on hand. It should preferably be transferred by means of a monthly standing order from the main partnership bank account, on a tax year basis so that for, say, the 1993/94 year, 12 monthly transfers would be made, from the end of April 1993 until March 1994.

A typical reserve is illustrated in Figure 26.3, which shows a four-doctor practice with an estimated liability for 1993/94 of £18 000. This could have been calculated in January or February 1993 and may require some amendment to take account of amended allowances and tax rates which have been introduced in the 1993 Budget. Interest will be credited to the various partners in proportions to their different contributions.

	Annual tax liability 1993/94 £	Monthly reserve April 1993–March 1994 £
Dr W	6000	495
Dr X	5000	410
Dr Y	4750	390
Dr Z	2250	185
	18 000	1480

The monthly transfer can be slightly less than $\frac{1}{12}$ of the annual liability, due to interest which will be credited to the account.

Figure 26.3   Income tax reserve

27 The Ownership of Surgeries

ONE of the factors that sets the NHS GP apart from other sections of the business community, including NHS dentists, is the manner in which the business premises are organized and financed. Detailed rules are contained in paragraph 51 of the SFA.

The provision of surgery premises is likely to fall under one of five categories:

1 rented from a private landlord
2 rented from the local authority
3 a health centre occupancy
4 owned by the partners
5 a cost rent development.

Some multi-surgery practices may have premises under two or more of these categories.

As discussed in Chapter 10, a relatively high level of GP expenses are refunded directly to the practice, and other expenses are refunded indirectly through the annual remuneration award. For surgery premises, however, a separate set of rules exist. It is necessary for GPs to understand these fully, as regards both rented and owner-occupied surgeries.

Rented surgeries

A GP who rents a surgery from a landlord has the right to recover the rent from the FHSA. Normally, this will be repaid fully, except in cases where the whole of the premises is not given over to NHS work. If, for instance, part of the property is sublet to a private tenant, a refund would not be made for that proportion of the rent. If the building is in combined use, partly for domestic or other use and the remaining part for the practice, an apportionment of the refund is normally calculated by the District Valuer.

Health centre accommodation

GPs practising from health centres should be aware that their rent (together with rates, water rates, etc) will not, in effect, be paid from their own sources and refunded, but will be internally recorded by the health authority.

In the case of both health centres and rented surgeries, care must be taken to see that the rent paid (or notional rent) is accurately shown on one side of the accounts and the (notional) refund on the other. This is to ensure that, if these accounts are selected by the Review Body for the 'sampling process', the GPs' expenses will be maximized so that they do not artificially depress the level of average expenses indirectly refunded in the annual pay award. This is particularly important for health centre practices, and the accountant drawing up the accounts should understand the necessity for this exercise.

In many cases, however, surgeries are not rented from a third party, but are owned by the doctor(s), either in sole practice or in partnership. In this case, a rent allowance is paid to the doctors in order to recompense them for the use of their privately-owned surgery for NHS purposes.

The notional rent allowance

Notional rent is paid on surgeries that are owner-occupied, but either are not new or have been erected or developed in a manner that falls outside the scope of the cost rent scheme (*see* Chapter 28). Notional rent payments for owner-occupiers, in respect of separate premises and/or premises forming part of a residence, are determined after assessment by the District Valuer according to a valuation based on the current market rent which may reasonably be expected to be paid for the premises.

The agreed amount is then paid in full to the GP(s), usually at quarterly or monthly intervals. Every effort should be made to improve cash flow (*see* Chapter 13) to ensure that the rent allowance is received monthly.

Notional rent is valued at triennial intervals, normally resulting in an increase in the rent allowance, and most practices show a steady increase in the rent allowance over the years. If they are not satisfied, the doctors have a right of appeal to the Secretary of State. This is frequently exercised and it is believed that, in the majority of cases, such appeals are successful. In some cases, however, due to the property recession, valuations have fallen. This is dealt with more fully in Chapter 29.

The community charge ('poll tax') is not property-related, and it cannot therefore be included in claims for refunds of direct expenses or personal expenses (*see* page 246). The new 'council tax', however, being a tax on property, can be included in such claims.

There are several other property-related reimbursements, which are dealt with in Chapter 10.

Cash limiting

With the introduction of new financial economies on the NHS, rent allowances and refunds (except notional rent) may be subject to cash limiting and financial cut-backs. GPs who are subject to such restrictions should seek to negotiate with their own FSHA, whose budgeting procedures are under local control.

Partnerships

The property-owning partnership is now extremely common, although many new surgery developments are only suitable or viable for larger group practices.

It is important to consider the effect of ownership on the organization of the practice finances.

It is common for such surgeries to be owned by the partners in other than their standard profit-sharing ratios. In a partnership of six doctors, two might be part-time or partially retired GPs who do not wish to partake in the surgery ownership, which would leave ownership in four shares.

The receipt of the cost or notional rent allowance, which is effectively the return on the partners' investment, should be credited to the surgery owners and not to the other partners. Similarly, the cost of servicing a loan should be dealt with on the same basis. This is illustrated in the accounts shown in Chapter 18, by the inclusion of separate notes (2 and 15) showing the allocation of such items as a prior share of profit.

See also Chapter 30: Capital Accounts.

Improvement grants

Grants are available for the improvement of surgery premises—currently up to a third of the total cost—although these are subject to 'cash limiting' by FHSAs in the same way as cost rent and other refunds.

Such grants are normally paid on completion of an improvement project, but improvements should only be embarked upon with the prior agreement of the FHSA.

One condition of claiming the improvement grant is that the same expenditure must not be claimed for income tax purposes. Whilst many improvements or alterations to the structure of the building will be of a capital nature and will not in any event attract capital allowances, there are certain circumstances in which tax relief could be claimed on identical expenditure, and a decision will have to be made as to which of these is preferable.

Whilst each case must be considered strictly on its individual merits, the present level of tax rates means that, for most such projects, it is more beneficial to claim the improvement grant and relinquish any potential tax relief.

Taxation

The rent allowance is paid to GPs on the use of privately owned surgeries to see NHS patients; it is unconnected with 'rent' in the generally accepted sense of the term, and it is essential that for taxation purposes this principle is understood. It is incorrect to treat the allowance as the private, unearned income of the doctor(s) and to enter it in the property section of their tax returns; otherwise this can have a radical effect both on the way the income is taxed and on the ultimate granting of retirement relief for capital gains tax on the eventual retirement of any of the joint owners.

The income should be treated as part of the practice profits, and allocated between the partners in ratios applicable to their shares of ownership for the property (not in those in which residual partnership profits are divided).

Relief for interest paid

Interest on surgery loans is allowed in full for tax purposes, and extreme care must be taken to see that only partners owning shares in the surgery premises obtain relief on the interest paid. Such relief is granted on the same basis that applies to all other expenses a GP incurs (*see* Chapter 38).

It is common, in cases of new surgery projects, for interest to be 'rolled up', ie not paid during the period of the surgery development but added to the loan for payment at a future date. This interest is also fully allowable on the same basis, but must be shown as an item of expenditure in the practice accounts. It may, however, be possible to re-organize the loan so that further tax benefit to the GP is made available (*see* Chapter 31),

New surgery developments

During recent years, most development projects have been financed under the cost rent scheme. Chapter 28 looks at how this operates and the advantages a GP can derive from it.

28 The Cost Rent Scheme

IN many cases during recent years, surgeries have been developed under a scheme introduced in the mid-1970s, which has provided new and vastly improved surgery accommodation for NHS patients.

The cost rent scheme offers a unique opportunity to acquire a valuable capital asset without significant capital outlay. No other profession, either inside or outside the NHS, is offered a scheme of a similar nature, the advantages of which are shown in Box 28.1.

Box 28.1: Benefits of the cost rent scheme

1 Tax-free capital appreciation.
2 Increasing income.
3 Taxation benefits.

Yet, surprisingly, many doctors have still not felt able to take advantage of it, in many cases being inhibited by the relatively large costs involved. This is unfortunate because the introduction of cash limiting from 1 April 1990 has in some cases succeeded in deferring or aborting new projects.

A concise account of the scheme, and the manner in which it operates, is given in *Making sense of the cost rent scheme*, published by Radcliffe Medical Press. This chapter looks at some of the implications for doctors embarking on a project for surgery development.

GPs who do not own their premises are eligible for reimbursement of the rent and rates paid on the premises, provided the FHSA is satisfied that the use of existing premises, the enlargement of premises, or a move to new premises, is justified in the interests of the NHS.

On the other hand, GPs who own their own premises are normally paid a rent allowance (as opposed to a refund) based upon the estimated rental value of the property. As an alternative to receiving a 'notional rent' reimbursement, however, some practices choose to apply for reimbursement related to the cost of providing purpose-built premises, or their equivalent. This is known as 'cost rent', provided that the project falls within one of the following categories:

1 the building of completely new premises
2 the acquisition of premises for substantial modification
3 the substantial modification of existing practice premises.

The scheme does *not* provide for the direct reimbursement of interest paid, or payable, on borrowing facilities arranged to meet the costs of a project; and it cannot be stressed too strongly that, before entering into a financial commitment or other obligation, GPs should ensure that the project is financially viable. They must be able to meet the costs of servicing and repaying the loan from the receipt of the cost rent allowance, other practice income and / or private means.

As the name implies, the cost rent scheme calculates the rent allowance by reference to the total cost of a development project, to which a percentage factor is applied. If, for instance, the total agreed cost of a project is £900 000, and there is a 7% fixed rate of cost rent in force at the time, the annual reimbursement will be £63 000.

There are four main components in the cost of such a project:

1 the cost of buying the land
2 the cost of erection (building contract)
3 professional and architects' fees
4 bridging interest.

With the imposition of cash limits on FHSAs, GPs should, at the outset of a project and before taking on any financial commitment, seek the FHSA's agreement to the proposals 'in principle', and ascertain the priority accorded to the project in the authority's forward programme for premises improvement, including any provisional estimate of when cost reimbursement can be expected for the scheme (SFA, paragraph 51.51). In other words, not only must approval be obtained for the project, but an indication must be given as to whether the FHSA is in a position to designate sufficient funds for the scheme and, if so, within which year's budget.

Detailed information must then be presented to the FHSA before a formal written offer will be issued which will:

1 confirm the acceptability of the project for cost rent reimbursement
2 set out the method to be used in calculating reimbursement
3 give a preliminary assessment of the level of reimbursement (the interim cost rent)
4 give a target date when the proposed reimbursement may take effect.

GPs must ensure that planning permission is obtained (or that it exists, or will be available), and that their architect is aware of the cost rent scheme and the limitations on size and building costs set out in paragraph 51.1 of the SFA. These limits are subject to regional variations in the form of four bands (*see* Appendix E), intended to reflect differences in building costs throughout the country. They are referred to in paragraph 51.3 of the SFA and are reviewed regularly and amended when necessary to keep in line with changes in building costs. Cost rent limits were, for instance, reduced by over 20% from June 1992, in order to take account of lower building costs.

Only those projects which are subject to a formal written offer and acceptance by the GPs of the terms thereof, will benefit from the banding increases, but it cannot be taken for granted that funds will be found within a particular FHSA's overall budget for a given year. Some projects may have to go on a waiting list in the hope of being accepted for inclusion in a later year's budget. Further, the FHSA's written offer will be conditional upon the project being completed within a given timescale; if without good reason the project cannot be completed within the specified time, then the authority may, at its discretion and without any obligation towards expenses to which the GPs have become committed, withdraw its approval. In such cases, the practitioners may find themselves out of pocket, with future expenses to meet, and will need to re-apply for cost rent reimbursement if they still wish to proceed.

FHSAs are under no obligation to increase the interim cost rent where the need for unforeseen additional works arise. In fact, the FHSA will almost invariably insist at the outset on fixed price building tenders. It is imperative that any changes to the GPs' plans for a project are advised to the FSHA immediately they occur, or are likely to occur.

Having found a suitable site for premises, GPs need to commission drawings, costings and building tenders, and apply for and obtain a formal written offer from the FHSA to gauge the level of cost rent reimbursement.

The cost rent limits

The maximum amount that may be spent on a new surgery project is strictly limited with respect to building costs. The current limits are set out in Appendix F on page 315.

Many developing practices have found it virtually impossible to build surgeries within these limits and have been left to finance a significant shortfall out of current earnings. This situation has to some degree been resolved by the introduction of variations in limits by means of the banding and other systems.

Location factors

From 1 June 1993, the system of four area bands was replaced by one based on building cost location factors applicable to each area in the UK. The factors currently in force are set out in Appendix E.

Total cost calculation

Once all the figures are available, it should be possible to establish with some degree of accuracy the likely level of cost rent reimbursement. Figure 28.1 shows a typical (if simplified) calculation for a practice in Berkshire to which a factor of 1.01 applies. It illustrates a typical situation where the proceeds from the cost rent allowance (£56 000) are identical to the interest on the loan finance, but not the annual cost of capital repayment.

This problem could be deferred by a capital repayment 'holiday' for the first few years of the loan, in the expectation that when capital repayments become due these will be covered by an increase in income due to a conversion to a 'notional rent' basis.

Fixed and variable allowances

Once the final cost rent limit has been calculated by the FHSA, the amount of cost rent reimbursement is calculated by applying to that limit the prescribed percentage as notified by the DoH to the authority. There are two percentage rates, one variable and the other fixed. The variable rate of reimbursement is reviewed annually in April (7% up to 31 March 1994), whereas the fixed rate of reimbursement (10% per annum at time of going to press) is set quarterly.

The variable rate of reimbursement is applied to every project *except* in the following circumstances when the fixed rate applies:

1 where GPs are financing the building scheme wholly or mainly with their own money
2 where they are financing it wholly or mainly with a loan acquired on fixed rate terms.

In both cases, either the input of the GPs' own monies or the draw-down of a fixed rate loan, must be for the majority of the total cost of the project.

		£	£
1	Site (cost or District Valuer's valuation, whichever is the lower)		120 000
2	Building cost (subject to cost rent limits) *Adjust*: for location factor (1.01)	475 000	
			479 750
			599 750
3	VAT @ 17.5% on £599 750 (see Chapter 43)		104 956
4	Architects' fees, etc VAT (17.5%)	55 171* 9655	
			64 826
5	Bridging interest		30 468
			800 000
	Cost rent reimbursement at variable rate (7%)		56 000

* Architects' fees at 11.5% of building cost + VAT.

Figure 28.1   Calculation of the cost rent allowance on a typical surgery development project

The SFA allows for situations where GPs finance the scheme wholly or mainly with a fixed rate loan, *but* with the option to switch to a variable rate at a future date. In such cases, the fixed rate of reimbursement will apply until the GP exercises the option and then the prevailing prescribed variable rate will be applied by the committee.

This ruling brings greater flexibility to the scheme and may be used to protect the GPs, or at least give them an advantage in times of rising interest rates. They can benefit from short-term fixed rate schemes made available by financial institutions, yet retain the ability to switch at a future date when there is a higher variable rate of reimbursement. The rate of reimbursement should be calculated by applying the approved prescribed percentage to the approved costs of the scheme; in the case of the variable rate, this is adjusted annually, but the fixed rate will not change regardless of general market conditions or rates.

Unless the aforementioned option is available, GPs should think carefully before committing themselves to borrowing at fixed rates. Long-term fixed rate borrowing may involve taking out an endowment policy and it should be asked whether the lending rate will be fixed for the duration of the loan. Thought should also be given to the situation of an incoming partner, who may be financially worse off by having a fixed rate of reimbursement, whilst having to borrow at a much higher variable rate to buy into a practice.

Advice should, at an early stage, be sought from the FHSA and the practice's financial advisers.

When to change to notional rent

Paragraph 51.52.21 of the SFA acknowledges that it is unlikely, initially, that the current market rate will produce a more favourable reimbursement than cost rent.

Cost rent will continue to be paid until the premises (or a significant part of them) cease to be used for practice purposes, or the GP chooses on a review to change to current market rent. A review can be requested:

1 every three years from the operative date of the cost rent when the premises are owned by the GPs, or
2 for premises leased by the GP, when a review of rent payable is due under the terms of the lease, or a new lease is entered into at the end of the full term of the existing lease.

Notional rent will be reviewed at triennial intervals after the switch from cost rent. No mention is made in the SFA of a reversal back to cost rent.

The decision to switch from cost rent to notional rent depends on several factors. Clearly, notional rent must exceed cost rent, and in the longer term the GP may feel relatively safe in the knowledge that property values and rents have, with few exceptions, risen each year. Nonetheless, at the time of the review consideration should be given, before authorizing the change-over, to the amount of the increased reimbursement compared with forecasts for interest rates, the economic and political climates, and the period to the next review of the prescribed variable rate. The benefit of a higher rate of notional rent reimbursement now would fade if, during the ensuing three years, the variable rate rose to dizzy heights as each annual review reflected rising rates in general.

In recent years, this factor has been influenced to some degree by a discernible trend towards reduction in notional rent assessments. This is discussed in detail in Chapter 29.

Raising the finance

Once the viability of the project has been established, FHSA approval obtained and other preliminaries concluded, funds will have to be raised to finance the project.

The cost rent is calculated according to a pre-determined formula, although this may be subject to some negotiation. The provision of the required loan and the agreement of interest and repayment rates are entirely separate issues, although the two must be compared when considering the net cost to the partners.

Arrangements must be made to obtain finance to purchase the site and to meet building and ancillary costs. Banks, insurance companies and the GP Finance Corporation may be prepared to provide surgery development finance at very competitive rates for periods of up to 20 or 25 years. Although a legal mortgage is taken over the surgery premises, and the land on which they stand, it is uncommon in the early years for the value of the land and buildings to equal or exceed the level of the corresponding loan facilities. The mortgage gives a degree of control to the lending institution in the event of, say, a partnership change or a default, but it could be argued that the real 'security' is the cost rent scheme and the reimbursements paid thereunder; these will continue for as long as the premises are deemed by the FHSA to be used for the purpose of GMS.

The lending institution must be satisfied that the GPs can service and repay the loan on the agreed terms because, in many cases, the cost rent reimbursement is lower than the amount required to service the debt, as FHSAs work to the lower of the actual building costs or the scheduled costs. Therefore, the GPs must be judged able to meet the cost of the shortfall between the cost rent allowance and a standing order to the lending institution. Unless the practitioners have private means, it is likely that the shortfall will be met from practice income. Although an analysis of the most recent balance sheets and accounts, FHSA quarterly returns and bank statements will be of considerable use, every practice is different in its circumstances and outlook.

In a group practice, it is important that this very real liability can be assessed at the outset by the individual GPs in the light of their needs and circumstances. This will have a bearing on whether they opt for an initial moratorium on capital repayments, an endowment-linked loan, a facility which is repaid by consecutive monthly instalments over the period agreed, or a combination of the three. There are advantages and disadvantages associated with all of these arrangements and, whilst many independent advisers prefer the flexibility of straight repayment (perhaps with an initial capital outlay), the important point is to work to what suits the individual's needs and best interests, rather than accept a rigid package of terms intended for universal application. Thought should also be given to the taking of a short-term life policy for each practitioner's share of the shortfall, although again this will depend on the individual circumstances and means.

The recession of the early 1990s has brought into play the further problem of negative equity, which is considered in detail in Chapter 29.

The final judgment

Any cost rent project must be judged essentially as a long-term investment. It is unlikely that any GP will realize a substantial benefit in the short term.

When all the information is available, a financial appraisal should be produced, which will give the GPs some idea of the likely surplus or shortfall. Figure 28.2 sets out a simplified version of such a statement.

	£	£
Total cost		800 000
Cost rent allowance (7% variable)		56 000
Loan repayments:		
Annual interest (7%)	56 000 (1)	
Capital repayments (25 years)	32 000	
		88 000
Total annual shortfall		32 000
Per partner (in a 6 partner practice)		5333

(1) Assumed to be 1% over bank base rate.

Figure 28.2   What will it cost (excluding taxation)?

29 The Problem of Negative Equity

FROM time to time a term enters our national consciousness which can cause such concern for those to whom it applies that one is bound to contemplate whether this represents a permanent change in our business ethos. One such term is 'negative equity', which has crept into common usage during the last few years, usually with regard to house owners, whose property has dropped in value to well below the amount of the loan originally taken out to buy the property. The house owner then cannot afford to sell the property, but will not be bankrupted if he keeps up his mortgage repayments.

No such comfort, however, awaits GPs who own their own surgeries. Negative equity is unlikely to be new to them, but they may, in the current recession, fail to prevent the situation from escalating. The prospect of the average practice continuing for even a few years without a change in partnership is rather remote and some highly unpopular decisions will normally have to be taken.

Sales and purchases between partners, of shares in a surgery, occur at fairly frequent intervals, but in the current economic situation these are likely to be affected by the problem of negative equity. GPs do, however, receive a direct reimbursement in the form of a cost or notional rent allowance, and this may pay the interest on the bank loan, and possibly part of the capital repayments. Therefore, even in a property recession, most owner-occupier GPs are able to service the loan from practice income.

The new surgery

GPs have, in the past, frequently experienced negative equity:

1 in developing new surgeries in urban areas, where building costs are likely to be high
2 where the development has lasted over a long period (entailing high bridging interest costs)
3 where there is a change of partnership shortly after completion, which necessitates a revaluation of the surgery.

Figure 29.1 shows a typical situation arising from a surgery development in 1988–9 with a total cost, including bridging interest, of £1.5 million.

A few months after the date of completion, the partnership decide to have the building valued, possibly for a change in partnership but probably for insurance purposes or to satisfy the bank that the security is still extant; the surgery is then valued at £1.1 million, yet the loan finance remains constant, giving an apparent negative equity of £400 000.

In many cases this will pose no undue problem to the practice. In a normal market, the value will increase again over the years, albeit from a lower base, so that when there is a partnership change, a retiring partner may be able to extract some equity from the sale of his surgery share.

The figure shows that the income position is by no means unsatisfactory; the partners are receiving cost rent of £172 500 against loan charges of £150 000, which gives an apparent surplus of £22 500. However, this assumes that the partners are making no capital repayments, probably through a moratorium arrangement, and that the surgery has been erected within the cost rent limits.

What then are the problems and what can be done about them? Where it is apparent that a partner in the practice is nearing retirement, it may not

Drs A, B & Partners

	Original finance K£	Position 31 December 1989 K£
Building Cost:		
Land etc	200	
Building costs	900	
Fees	150	
	1250	–
Valuation	–	1100
Bridging Interest	250	–
		1100
Loan Finance	(1500)	(1500)
Negative Equity		(400)

BUT Income position:	£
Cost rent (11.5% on £1.5 mil)	172 500
Interest on loan (10% variable)	150 000
Surplus	22 500

Figure 29.1   Negative equity resulting from a new surgery development completed 1 June 1989

be beneficial for him to become involved in the surgery development, as it may not be possible for him to acquire a reasonable level of equity in the few remaining years. A partner may easily be excluded from ownership of the building and consequent liability to repay the mortgage. This merely requires the partnership accounts to be designed in such a manner as to reflect this position in the allocation of income and expenses between the partners.

Some partnerships, if well advised, have been able to see this problem in advance, and have inserted a clause in the partnership deed to say that the building may not be sold for less than cost. Consequently, if a partner retires, he would not be left with a liability, nor would he have acquired any equity: there would therefore be no such payment to him on his retirement, but neither would he be asked to make any contribution. However, there might be the problem of a construed sale of goodwill.

Where this clause does not apply, practices may find themselves in the embarrassing position of having to approach a retiring partner and ask him to introduce funds to make up his share of the negative equity. The second column of Figure 29.1 shows a negative equity of £400 000. Assuming this is a four-doctor practice, with all partners owning the surgery equally, a retiring partner may be asked to contribute £100 000 on his retirement.

All practices which are liable to find themselves in this situation are strongly advised either to exclude a senior partner from such a development or to include a clause, to the effect outlined above, in their partnership deed.

The new partner

The above solution, while it may satisfy the requirements of an outgoing partner, is unlikely to entirely satisfy those of the continuing surgery owners, or particularly a new partner who is asked to buy into the equity of the building.

The continuing partners will be obliged to purchase a one-quarter share of the building from their retiring colleague. If one excludes the balance of the outstanding loan, each of the three will, in the example (Figure 29.1), have paid £125 000 (one-third of £375 000) for a one-twelfth share which, on the current valuation, is worth £91 667 (leaving a deficit of £33 333). Whilst they will have financed this additional purchase, presumably by taking out an additional loan, they will at least have the comfort of each receiving one-third of the cost rent allowance, rather than the quarter received before the date of change. They can also, depending on the vagaries of the property market, look forward to an appreciation in value in the long term.

The above assumes that an outgoing surgery-owning partner will be bought out by his colleagues. However, in some cases outgoing partners retain their share in the surgery for up to a year, and then sell directly to an incoming partner who may by then have served a probationary period or have progressed at least part of the way to parity. Where a sale is made directly to the continuing partners, they may continue to own the surgery between them or they may pass on, at some time in the future, a quarter share to the incoming partner.

Whichever of these apply, given the current situation an incoming partner is likely to face significant problems, both in buying his share and in justifying the price asked. In our example, it is assumed that the incoming partner will be expected to pay the price paid to the outgoing partner, ie £375K (one-quarter of £1500K), despite the fact that the true value is only £275K (one-quarter of £1100K). He may well jib at being asked to meet such a price for a property which is, on current valuations, grossly over-valued—why should he not seek to take advantage of the depressed property market? There is no easy answer, although some practices have sought to resolve this by agreeing to sell to the incoming partner at the up-to-date valuation, with the continuing partners carrying the loss between them. Again, the goodwill question should also be borne in mind.

The only real alternative is for the new partner not to buy into the surgery at all. However, this sets an unfortunate precedent which can apply on successive changes until only one doctor owns the building. What will happen when he wants to retire?

Some practices put pressure upon partners to buy in at the orginal (possibly cost) price, in the knowledge that this is in excess of the true valuation, but with the security that the cost rent income is based upon the original cost.

Existing surgeries

Figure 29.2 shows a rather different situation of an inner city practice which has owned the surgery for many years. This was revalued on a partnership change in 1989 at £650K, and that amount has been used in the practice balance sheet since that date. The practice has an endowment mortgage with a major clearing bank of £600K. This will ultimately be repaid by means of endowment policies on the lives of two partners, but this is of comparatively recent origin and there is no significant surrender value in these policies. However, at that date the practice had an equity in the building of £50K and, after receiving cost rent and servicing the loan interest, the two virtually balanced.

Drs W, X and Y

	1988 position K£	1993 position K£
Valuation 31 December 1989	650	
31 January 1993		350
Loan Finance	600	600
Positive equity, 1989	50	
Negative equity, 1993		250

Figure 29.2 Negative equity on an existing surgery which is revalued in 1989, and from which a partner retires on 31 January 1993

However, the new senior partner, Dr W, announced his intention to retire at the end of January 1993, and to sell his share in the surgery to his partners on the same date. The partners obtained separate valuations of the surgery at £350K, which was in accordance with current values in the area. The outstanding loan remained unchanged over the period, so that the negative equity had reached £250K.

To make matters even more difficult, Dr Y, who joined as a junior partner on 1 January 1990, did not reach parity until 1 January 1993, from which date he was given an option to buy a one-third share of the surgery. However, in view of the valuation of the outstanding loan, he decided not to buy a share of the building, and the ownership therefore devolved on Dr X alone, who was due to retire three years later.

Although there was no relevant clause in the partnership deed, Drs W and X between them agreed that Dr W would be paid out on the basis of the amount outstanding under the loan, which gave him nil equity. Dr X was subsequently left with the outstanding loan, the interest on which was more or less covered by the rent allowance received. Dr X is unlikely to be able to attract new partners to buy the surgery from him on this basis and will struggle to repay the loan on his retirement.

He is now in a classic 'no win' situation. Whilst he remains in practice, he will be able to make the interest payments, but the combined endowment premiums must be met out of his personal income. It is essential that he make a decision within three years, and his only options appear to be:

1 to sit tight and hope that the property market picks up
2 at age 57, to defer his plan to retire when he reaches 60-years-old

3 to retire and seek to charge an enhanced rent for the practice (but he has no assurance that his continuing partners will be able or prepared to pay such a higher rent, particularly if it results in a CGT disadvantage)
4 to sell the building for what he can get, repay the mortgage, cash in the insurance policy and meet the deficit out of his own personal estate, if indeed such funds are available.

Many older GPs are now finding themselves in this situation. The mere ownership of an NHS surgery no longer ensures the property-owning partner of a handsome tax-free nest egg on retirement. Some partners, who acquired property at a lower value in the early stages of their careers, are still sitting on such profits, but these are becoming fewer.

Whilst there is no easy answer to such a problem, specialist advice should be sought in order to make a logical decision.

Notional rent allowance

In recent years, District Valuers, on revaluing surgeries for the purposes of notional rent assessment, have sometimes regraded them downwards. This has happened in many parts of the country; if prevailing rents in an area fall, the District Valuer must take account of this.

Needless to say, practices which find themselves in such a position are strongly advised to appeal against the reassessment. For example, a practice which has for some years received a rent allowance of £27 000, and is provisionally reassessed at £19 000 (a fall of some 30%), should certainly appeal.

GPs in this situation should consult paragraph 51, Schedule 4(2)[a][i]) of the SFA, which provides for a basis of assessment for owner-occupied premises on the assumption of a lease of 15 years and upwardly assessed reviews every three years. Although the definition is rather ambiguous, the implication is that reviews may only be made upwards, and never downwards.

Other partnership changes

The problem of negative equity can restrict changes in partnerships which would otherwise be desirable. Practices may be unable to recruit new partners for the reasons discussed in this chapter. Conversely, a practice wishing to dispose of the services of a partner may feel inhibited from doing so if it becomes apparent that this will result in the departing partner being required to pay, say, £100 000 into the practice in respect of his share of the negative equity.

There is also the vexed question of goodwill to be considered. The sale and purchase of goodwill in NHS practices is illegal, including the sale of assets at an inflated value. If, therefore, a new partner is asked to pay £150 000 for a share of surgery premises which is generally acknowledged to be worth £120 000, is the extra £30 000 a hidden sale of goodwill? The latest interpretations by the MPC indicate that this is the case and that a GP knowingly involved in such a transaction acts illegally.

Ownership by trust

Some practices have sought to avoid the above dilemma by transferring the property into a form of trust, so that the building is owned by the practice in perpetuity, rather than by the individual partners holding shares. For practices which already have a severe problem, it may well be too late for this to be an effective solution, but practices currently bringing new surgeries into use may find such an arrangement to be beneficial.

30 Capital Accounts

THERE is no single matter concerning the finances of the medical partnership which causes such consternation and misunderstanding as the concept of capital accounts and the contributions incoming partners are required to make. Despite the regular stream of articles in the medical press, explaining various aspects of capital accounts, there remains a significant lack of understanding on the part of young partner who may regard himself as still an employee, either of the health authority or the practice, and fail to realize the concept of investment in a business and of the returns to be made from it.

This concept of investment in the capital of the business is not confined to medical practices. A multinational company needs to raise capital, to develop its potential and finance its current operations, and this is normally done through share issues or loans from banks or finance houses. GPs running a practice, often with a turnover in excess of £1 million a year, must also finance their business operations, surgery development and numerous items of capital equipment, furniture etc, required to run the practice.

There are two sources of finance available to the GP: loans from outside sources (a bank, GPFC etc) or personal resources—either private funds, which may have been borrowed, or restrictions of future drawings. It is more efficient in financial terms if capital comes from the personal resources of the partners rather than from constant and expensive borrowing from the bank, unless it is absolutely necessary.

The various components of capital are shown in Box 30.1 and are discussed in this chapter.

Box 30.1: The capital of a medical partnership: components

1 Property capital: net equity in surgery buildings.
2 Other (fixed asset) capital: investment in furniture, fixtures, fittings, equipment, computers, office machinery, etc.
3 Working capital: the net current assets of the practice.

2 and 3 can be simplifed to fixed capital.

Property (or surgery) capital

This applies to surgery-owning practices only. In the case of the financing of surgery developments or the acquisition of shares of equity by a new partner, the money involved will normally be financed by outside sources of borrowing (*see* surgery ownership, Chapter 27). The initial investment by the GPs will be quite small. Indeed, in many surgery projects, there is 100% financing from the bank. However, the partners' contribution will tend to increase with time due to appreciation in property values and through capital repayments of the loan.

The situation arising upon the retirement of an outgoing partner and the introduction of a new partner, where it is proposed to make a sale from the retiring to the incoming partner, is shown in Figure 30.1. The practice developed a new surgery in 1986 at a cost of £250 000, which was wholly borrowed so that there was no initial contribution by the partners. The first change in ownership took place in 1993; the valuation had increased to £400 000, with the loan having been partially repaid and standing at £210 000. This established the equity in the surgery building at £190 000, which is the basis upon which all calculations should be made. The outgoing partner has a one-fifth share from which he would reasonably expect to receive a sum of £38 000. An incoming partner should expect to contribute on the same basis. It can be seen from this example how equity has built up over this seven-year period.

	1986 £	1993 £
Original cost, 1986	250 000	
Valuation: 31 March 1993		400 000
Less: balance of outstanding loan	250 000	210 000
Equity	–	190 000
One-fifth share	–	38 000
Equity has built up due to:		
Surplus on revaluation (£400K – £250K)		150 000
Part repayment of loan (£250K – £210K)		40 000
		190 000

Figure 30.1   Surgery capital: calculation of partnership share

One aspect of surgery capital, which is represented by the equity in the surgery building, is that it is frequently owned by the partners in different proportions to those in which they share practice profits. In a typical partnership, there may be six partners, one of whom is a partially retired GP who has sold his share of the surgery, and another a part-time doctor who is unable to buy a share; the four remaining partners own the surgery, possibly equally, although this may not be the same means by which they share profits from the practice.

In medical partnerships, this causes no undue problems of principle; the proceeds from the surgery ownership, which in practice will be the notional or cost rent allowance together with any other small rentals the practice might receive, less the interest and the surgery loan should be credited to the surgery-owning partners. It is normal to deal with this by inclusion of a separate allocation in the annual accounts (*see* page 102). Only by this means can the surgery-owning partners receive the correct return on their investment in the surgery premises, as opposed to their colleagues who have made no such contribution.

In recent years, the term 'negative equity' has come into use to denote the situation applying where the loan on a surgery building is higher than the current valuation. This is considered at some length in Chapter 29.

Other (fixed asset) capital

Apart from the surgery, there will almost certainly be additional capital assets employed by the practice, which it is necessary to record as capital in the books of the partnership and which the partners can expect to exchange among themselves for value on changes in either the constitution of the partnership or in profit-sharing ratios.

These assets will normally consist of items owned by the practice as a whole: furniture (desk, chairs, tables, filing cabinets, etc); fixtures and fittings (heating installations, plumbing fittings, fixed shelving and filing areas, etc); medical and surgical equipment (X-ray machines, etc); office machinery and equipment (telephone installations, computers, copying machines, etc). In a sizeable practice this could add up to several thousand pounds, and it is normal for a retiring partner to take his share of this on retirement and for the incoming partner to purchase a share of it.

Unlike the surgery building, the return from these assets cannot be quantified exactly; they are, in effect, assets from which the practice earns its income and profits, so that it is reasonable for such assets to be divided in the same ratios as those in which the partners share practice profits.

It is normal for a valuation to be taken when changes in partnership occur. If, for instance, a value of £5000 was placed on fixed assets, the retiring partner could reasonably expect to receive a one-fifth share, ie £1000. However, an incoming partner may not be asked to contribute to the same degree if entering at a lower ratio, say 12%, and moving to parity over several years. At 12%, his contribution would only be £600. The remainder should be contributed, normally by drawings adjustments, over the period to parity.

Working capital

The concept of working capital, normally represented by the net current assets of the partnership, is probably the most difficult for incoming partners to understand. Working capital involves less obvious assets, such as those held in cash and debts due to the practice. New partners frequently express surprise when they are asked to contribute to these current assets, although they are part of the legitimate capital of the business from which they earn their income.

In Figure 30.2, the working capital requirement at a given date of a dispensing practice is shown as net current assets of £50 000. At any given date, the practice may be required to hold a fairly large stock of drugs; there may at times be substantial funds due to the practice from the FHSA and other sources, which it must finance from its own means; and there will be amounts owed by the practice to outside creditors, probably for drug supplies, etc. An incoming partner commencing on a starting share of 12% of the profits could reasonably expect to pay in the same proportion of that amount, ie £6000. In the case of a large dispensing practice, it is normal for this to be done by an initial introduction of funds, at the same time as the fixed assets are purchased. In the case of a smaller practice with a reduced capital requirement, the partners may be prepared to accept a gradual build-up of funds due to the restrictions of drawings over an agreed period.

Retiring partners

For partners retiring from practice, who wish to recover the capital invested by them in the practice, the process is relatively easy with respect to the

Current assets:	£
Stock of dispensing drugs	40 000
Sundry debtors	25 000
Cash at bank	2500
Cash in hand	50
	67 550
Less: Sundry creditors	17 550
Net current assets	50 000

Figure 30.2   Working capital: net current assets

surgery and other capital. Valuations are placed on the assets and the gross value or equity calculated. The calculation of the working capital normally has to wait until the next partnership accounts are prepared so that the amount can be accurately assessed. The partnership deed should lay down in strict terms the manner in which this capital is to be paid over to a retiring partner or the executors of a deceased partner.

Where fixed capital amounts are in operation, the process is a great deal easier, as retiring partners are then fully aware of the extent of their capital investment.

Goodwill

The sale and purchase of goodwill in NHS general practices is illegal and is prohibited under the National Health Service Act. Unlike their colleagues in the dental services, NHS GPs are not deemed to hold any value of goodwill and it cannot be passed, either in specific terms or as 'hidden goodwill', upon changes in partnership. GPs held to have taken part in such transactions can be treated severely by the medical authorities, including the General Medical Council.

This prohibition on the sale and purchase of goodwill does not apply to private practices, which are able to transact such business without hindrance.

Fixed capital accounts

Some partnerships express a preference for having their capital calculated on a fixed sum, intended to represent their investment in both the fixed assets and working capital of the practice. This system has a number of advantages.

1 By more exactly quantifying the required capital investment by each partner, it facilitates the introduction of new partners.
2 For similar reasons, it is easier to calculate the capital due to an outgoing partner.
3 It ensures that the balances on the partners' current accounts at the end of the year represent undrawn profits which can be paid over to them.
4 It facilitates the organization of loan finance to provide the most tax-efficient result for each partner. This is discussed more fully in Chapter 31.

It is normal for these fixed capital amounts to be allocated between partners in profit-sharing ratios. Thus, whilst the overall level of capital might not change, the allocation between individual partners may be changed in accordance with revised profit-sharing ratios, eg when a junior partner progresses to parity.

From the amounts set out in Chapter 18, the balance sheet (page 101) indicates that the overall fixed capital has been set at £80 000. The allocations between individual partners (Note 21) are equivalent to their shares of the profit.

31 Efficient Capital Planning

ON numerous occasions, GPs, as partners in their businesses, are required to fund fairly large capital contributions, and this chapter examines how partners can:

1 organize the capital of their practice in such a way that it will remain constant from year to year (and how this figure can be calculated)
2 re-organize a substantial surgery mortgage to maximize tax benefits
3 re-organize their private loan arrangements to 'unlock' some or all of the capital, again for tax benefit.

Fixed capital accounts

We have seen in Chapter 30 (page 186) how some partnerships can re-organize their capital in such a manner that a fixed sum is quantified, which represents an investment by the partners in the fixed assets and working capital of the practice. Page 187 sets out the advantages in doing so.

In the specimen practice accounts on pages 98–112, the balance sheet (page 101) shows the overall fixed capital of the practice at £80 000. This is calculated by adding to the written value of the fixed assets (excluding the surgery) shown in the balance sheet, the total required working capital of the partnership. Figure 31.1 illustrates this; it takes into account the fixed assets (£59 264) together with the stock and debtors, and deducts from these the current liabilities to arrive at £66 895. Added to this figure is the estimated amount the partners require to run the practice on a day to day basis for the ensuing month. Most practices receive money on a regular monthly basis and can fairly accurately estimate the amount required to meet all known expenses during a typical month. This figure has been calculated at £13 000. The total figure arrived at by this process is £79 895, rounded up for ease of accounting to £80 000, which will remain constant unless there are significant variations in ensuing years, such as a substantial investment by the partners in fixed assets, which will greatly increase the total.

Having established how the practice's capital can be estimated, use can be made of the knowledge to organize the capital on the loans taken out to finance it, in a way which gives the partners the maximum possible tax advantage.

	£	£
Fixed assets (at written-down value)		59 264
Current assets:		
Stock	4275	
Debtors	12 946	
	17 221	
Less: Due to former partner	(948)	
Sundry creditors	(8642)	7631
		66 895
Cash requirement (on monthly basis)		13 000
Fixed capital requirement		79 895
(rounded)		80 000

Figure 31.1   Calculation of fixed capital requirement at 30 June 1993

Re-financing surgery loans

GPs are taxed on a self-employed basis under Schedule D, which means that profits earned for, say, the year ending 30 June 1992 will be assessed for tax in the 1994–5 tax year, so that the tax will be payable over a year after the profits are earned.

One major advantage of this is that it defers tax liability on total income, although by the same token tax is also relieved on expenditure in the same period a year afterwards. It would be more beneficial if a system could be introduced whereby the delay in payment of tax would apply to income, but not to expenditure.

In any surgery-owning partnership, a major item of expenditure is the interest on the loan originally taken out on the surgery development. It is normal for such loans to be taken out on a partnership basis, so that the interest is passed through the partnership accounts and effectively relieved for tax a year later. This principle also extends to interest which was 'rolled up' during the period of development before the surgery was occupied. It is essential that the tax relief attracted by this loan is not only properly organized, but is maximized (*see* page 166).

GPs can also make use of the present tax law to obtain top rate tax relief on interest paid on a loan taken out to introduce capital into the partnership. By this means, the partnership's surgery loan might be repaid, from taking out individual loans which are injected into the partnership and effectively replace the original borrowing. The beauty of the scheme is that it transfers the effect of tax relief from a preceding year to an actual year basis, so that surgery-owning doctors obtain such relief a year earlier than would otherwise be the case. Moreover, at the outset, the doctors get a double tax benefit for up to 21 months from the date of the change. Figure 31.2 shows how this works.

Referring to the accounts set out in Chapter 18, the practice owns a surgery at a book value of £631 471, which is secured upon a long-term mortgage of £426 426 (*see* Note 21, page 109) with the Branshire Bank PLC. Note 20 (page 109) tells us that the property is owned by four partners only, and on page 107 (Note 15) we see that during the year the practice paid £40 264 in loan interest against a charge of £48 697 in the year 30 June 1992, the fall presumably arising from lower interest rates during the second period.

Let us then say that, on 1 July 1993, the partnership repaid that surgery loan by drawing a cheque for the amount outstanding and paying this to the lending bank involved. This entailed a substantial overdrawing on the partnership bank current account for a limited period, which would have required the knowledge and agreement of the bank. At the same time, the four surgery-owning partners agreed with their bank to take out separate loans in their own names for the purpose of introducing capital into the partnership. Provided they maintained that the loan was for this reason, the partners should have had no undue difficulty in obtaining the consequent tax relief. In this case, each of the four partners took out a personal loan of £106 106.50 (a quarter of £424 426).

Figure 31.2 shows how the partners will benefit to the sum of £11 000 in the year 1993–4 and £16 000 in 1994–5. During those years double taxation relief will be received, on the one hand on the preceding basis by passing the interest through the partnership accounts, and on the other on the actual year basis on the loans taken out for introduction of capital. In succeeding years this double relief will cease, but the benefit of relief on an actual year basis will continue, so greatly improving the cash flow position of the practice.

In summary, the benefits that accrue from this process are as follows.

1 Tax relief will be transferred onto an actual year basis.
2 'Double' tax relief will be obtainable for a limited initial period.
3 As a result of the forthcoming introduction of a new system of taxing the self-employed, which will abolish the preceding year basis, (*see* Chapter 38, page 225), in the transitional period it is likely that one year's profits will fall out a charge to tax. If re-financing on the lines set out above is not arranged, one year's cost rent income will escape tax, but tax relief will

	1993/94 £	1994/95 £
Per partnership accounts:		
Tax relief on preceding year basis:		
£48 697 @ 40%	19 479	
£40 264 @ 40%		16 106
Tax relief on actual year basis:		
1 July 1993 to 5 April 1994		
£30 000 @ 40%	12 000	
6 April 1994 to 5 April 1995		
£40 000 @ 40%		16 000
Total relief	31 479	32 106
Less: originally granted on preceding year basis	19 479	16 106
	12 000	16 000
Less: continued costs of transfer	1000	
Net saving	11 000	16 000

Figure 31.2   Re-financing of surgery loans, assuming transfer of mortgages on 1 July 1993

also be lost on one year's interest. By re-financing, the cost rent will still escape a charge to tax but there will be no loss of tax relief on the interest paid.

4 Where partners wish to make private pension contributions, which depend on the level of profits assessable for the tax year, relevant income upon which pension relief will be granted will be proportionately greater.

Before going ahead with such a scheme, the property-owning partner should, however, be aware of a number of potential problems.

(i)   Care should be taken to ensure that there is no overriding penalty on the redemption of an existing partnership loan. Some lending organizations have tried to impose harsh conditions where such loans are repaid, not only charging penalties but seeking to impose undue restrictions on the personal loans which succeed it.

(ii)   An arrangement fee may be charged by the bank for taking out each new loan. In addition, there may be a charge for legal fees, which should be avoided if possible.

(iii) A lending institution will wish to secure the borrowings. As the loans are in the personal names of the individual partners, it will be necessary for cross guarantees to be given so that if, say, a partner dies in service or retires, the bank has the security of knowing that his loan continues to be covered.

(iv) Detailed arrangements should be made to cover the eventuality of partners leaving or retiring from practice. This may necessitate an amendment to the partnership deed.

Tax-efficient borrowing

Many partners have outstanding loans upon which they gain either no tax relief or relief restricted to the basic rate. Such loans may have been those taken out to cover excessive personal spending, or to pay school fees or a house mortgage in excess of £30 000. Overdrafts and borrowings on credit cards are other examples of borrowings which are inefficient for tax purposes.

It is possible to repay these inefficient borrowings and replace them by loans which carry tax relief at the highest rate, as shown in Figure 31.3. This is normally commenced by the partner arranging for his bank to set up a new personal loan account, taken out entirely for the purpose of introducing capital into the partnership. Once this principle has been established, the partner can then draw a cheque on the partnership account up to the amount of his borrowing, and use this to repay loans which do not attract tax relief. He will then draw down the borrowing on the new personal loan arrangement with his bank and use it to replenish his capital account by paying the cheque into the partnership. It is essential that these transactions are completed in the correct sequence, and that the bank manager's co-operation is obtained in advance.

This process can be implemented by one or more partners in a practice; other partners who may not wish, or have no need, to participate need not do so.

It must again be strongly emphasized that the extent of the benefit which a partner can obtain by this means is limited to the amount of his capital investment in the practice. This will be apparent from a glance at the practice accounts which will show the amount outstanding on his capital account. There is little point, for instance, in a partner with a capital balance of £5000 seeking to take out a loan of, say, £20 000. This would almost certainly result in the tax relief not being granted and the partner will effectively have lost the cost of fees in setting up the new arrangement, without any consequent benefit. Moreover, the capital account balance should not go below the amount borrowed, or tax relief will again be lost.

Dr Green, who has an agreed level of investment of £17 600 in the fixed capital of his partnership, wishes to re-finance this in order to repay borrowings on which no tax relief is being received

	£
Personal overdraft	4000
School fees loan	8000
Credit card borrowings	3500
Loan for house extension (1991)	4500
	20 000

He negotiates with his bank manager a new personal loan of £17 600, for the purpose of introducing capital into the partnership, at an interest rate of 1.5% over base, secured on his share of the partnership capital. He cannot borrow the full £20 000 as this is above the level of his capital balance.

He then draws a cheque for £17 600 on the partnership account, with the agreement of his partners, and uses this to repay the latter three loans (£16 000 in all), with the balance of £1600 being set against his overdraft. The following day he draws the full amount of his new loan, so replenishing the partnership account. This will enable him to receive tax relief as follows:

	£
Interest (pa) on £17 600 at 7.5%	1320
Tax relief at 40%	528

Figure 31.3 How to transfer borrowings to obtain maximum tax relief (based on specimen practice accounts in Chapter 18)

Where a partner already has personal borrowings, either in respect of the surgery or other partnership capital, he can still increase his borrowings if there is capital equity remaining. For this purpose, and provided a realistic valuation is used, he must first repay all relevant borrowing and then take out an entirely new loan for the larger amount.

These processes are extremely complex and it is emphasized that they should only be carried out following knowledgeable professional advice.

32 Training Practices

SOME practices are authorized to employ GP trainees during their vocational training period. Only GPs who have undergone a three-year vocational training period are allowed to join practices as principals, and young doctors who propose to enter general practice must therefore comply with these requirements.

In this chapter, the financial arrangements that apply to the trainer and trainee are considered.

It is normal for at least one GP in a partnership to be appointed a trainer. In larger partnerships, two or more trainees may be engaged simultaneously, provided the requisite number of partners have been approved as trainers. In financial terms, the trainer receives a trainee supervision grant as recompense for the work involved, whilst the practice receives reimbursement from the FHSA for the trainee's salary and other payments made on his behalf.

It is important that the refund received from the FHSA matches the amount paid to the trainee (*see* Figure 32.1). In legal and taxation terms, the trainee is an employee of the trainer (or of his partnership), who is legally accountable to the Inland Revenue for tax under the PAYE regulations and Class 1 National Insurance contributions.

Some FHSAs calculate the trainee refund on a quarterly basis; in these cases, the practice should ensure that monthly paytments on account are received to maintain good cash flow.

	Paid by practice (monthly) £		Recovered from FHSA £
Recovered from FHSA: gross salary			2144 (2)
Net salary to trainee (1)		1600	
Paid to Collector of Taxes: PAYE	400 (3)		
Class 1 NIC:			
Employer	166 (4)		166 (4)
Employee	144 (5)	710	
		2310	2310

(1) Net salary calculated (gross):

Less:	Tax (3)	400		(2) 2144
	NIC (5)		144	544
				(1) 1600

Figure 32.1 The GP trainee: salary refund August 1993

Income tax

The practice should operate PAYE on the employee's salary, including London weighting where appropriate, and any other increments that may apply, including the trainee car allowance (*see* page 196) and any other amount that might be paid to the trainee above his normal salary.

Income tax need not be applied to refunds of expenditure, such as telephone charges, removal expenses and defence society subscriptions.

National Insurance

The trainee salary is fully chargeable to Class 1 NIC under the normal rules in force and using tables supplied to the employer. These should be applied at the contracted-out rate, but see page 196 for separate NIC rules applying to the trainee car allowance.

Trainee's superannuation

On the FHSA remittance statement to the practice, 6% of the trainee's salary is deducted in respect of superannuation contributions. More may be deducted if the trainee is buying added years. The practice must ensure that these deductions are recovered from the trainee's salary before payment, otherwise the trainer and the practice will be out of pocket. Superannuation should be deducted from the gross pay before the PAYE tax is calculated, but it is not deductible when calculating Class 1 NIC.

The trainee supervision grant

The trainee supervision grant is paid to the trainer as part of the remuneration for services as a trainer. This should be allocated in accordance with the wishes of the partners as set out in the partnership deed and displayed in the annual accounts. In some practices, this will be retained by the trainer personally; in most cases, it will be aggregated with partnership profits for division.

Superannuation at the trainer's own rate (standard plus added years if applicable) is deducted from the supervision grant on payment by the FHSA, and this should be charged in the partnership current accounts to the trainer concerned, unless election has been made to the FHSA for it to be allocated in partnership ratios.

Other payments and refunds

Occasionally, various payments will be made to the trainer by way of refund from the FHSA in respect of payments made by the trainee. These should be passed on to whoever has made the original payment. For instance, payments made in part reimbursement of defence society subscriptions by the trainee should be passed on to him. If reimbursements are made, the trainee can claim tax relief only on the net amount after deduction of the refund.

Removal expenses may well have originally been paid by the trainee and should also be paid over to him. No tax is chargeable if these are genuine reimbursements. Similarly, with regard to refunds of telephone rentals, if the original bills were paid by the practice then the refund should be paid into the partnership account.

The trainee car allowance

The trainee car allowance and the means by which it should be taxed cause much controversy.

Under strict tax law, this allowance is part of the trainee's salary; it is paid as part of his contract with the NHS and is properly assessable to income tax. However, provided certain procedures are applied, relief can be obtained for some or all of the amount paid. It is suggested that the following procedure is adopted, in order of preference shown below.

1 The PAYE tax district of the practice should be approached to obtain a general clearance for the trainee car allowance to be paid to the trainee without deduction of tax. If this is accepted by the Inspector of Taxes, the problem is largely solved, for the practice if not for the trainee.

   Once obtained, clearance normally applies to successive trainees and will not have to be re-applied for when a new trainee is engaged. The allowance should merely be paid over to the trainee by adding one-twelfth of the annual rate of allowance to his salary, there being no need to operate the PAYE system.

   Some tax districts are not prepared to give this clearance, and we must then look at the next stage.

2 The trainee should be asked to approach his own tax district (normally the district dealing with the PAYE affairs of the practice) and ask for an increase to his code number to take account of the car allowance. If this is provided, the trainer can operate the PAYE system using the higher coding. This will give the same result as if the clearance outlined above had been granted.

3 If points 1 and 2 are both unacceptable to the tax district, the only alternative is for the trainer, for his own and his practice's protection, to deduct tax from the trainee on the whole of the car allowance as well as his salary, using the code number he is given. It must be emphasized that the negotiation of such a code number is the responsibility of the trainee and not of the employer.

If this situation applies, it is likely that the trainee can obtain a refund at the end of the year, provided it can be demonstrated clearly to the Inspector of Taxes that the money has been spent on running the car for the use of the practice. This will normally be done using generally accepted principles (*see* Chapter 42).

It is convenient for claims of this nature by GP trainees to be submitted using Inland Revenue form P87.

It must be emphasized that the responsibility for deducting tax and National Insurance from the trainee car allowance lies with the employer (the trainer). If the Inland Revenue finds that he has not operated tax according to the rules in force, large sums of unpaid tax covering several years could be due from the trainer.

Trainees should approach their PAYE tax office for local rulings as to the charging of Class 1 National Insurance contributions on the trainee car allowance.

33 Dispensing Practices

A minority of NHS practices are permitted to dispense drugs and appliances to their own patients. Recent statistics show that this involves some 3650 GPs throughout the UK, representing about 11% of doctors in NHS practices. The dispensing facility leads to a number of accounting problems.

For the accounting year 1990/91, payments to dispensing GPs accounted for some £193 million, which was 24% of NHS direct re-reimbursements totalling £816 million. This excludes dispensing fees and oncosts, yet is the second largest single refund after staffing payments. Governments wishing to control public spending have therefore concentrated much of their efforts on trying to limit expenditure under this heading.

Generally, in order to qualify as a dispensing practice and be accepted under the scheme, patients for whom the dispensing facility is made available should reside more than one mile from the nearest pharmacist. This usually limits dispensing practices to rural and a few suburban areas: those areas in the UK which have the greatest proportion of dispensing practices are Lincolnshire and North Yorkshire (each 52%). There is continuing controversy between dispensing doctors and the pharmacists' associations over the right to dispense, as on the one hand GPs' dispensing facilities give a greatly increased level of service to patients, and on the other hand they can deprive qualified pharmacists (who might give a better service) of their livelihood.

Detailed regulations for the calculation of reimbursements to dispensing doctors are contained in paragraph 44 of the SFA. This stipulates that the payments should be calculated under six separate headings.

1 The basic price, calculated in accordance with the group tariff currently in force. From this price an average figure is deducted for estimated discount, which is discussed further below.
2 An oncost allowance of 10.5% of the basic price before the deduction of such a discount.
3 A container allowance of 3.8p per prescription.
4 A dispensing fee, which is on a sliding scale, according to the number of scrips issued per month.
5 An addition in respect of VAT at the rate currently in force.
6 Any exceptional expenses provided for by the drug tariff.

Profitability

Many dispensing practices are highly profitable. The level of profit earned from dispensing depends on the efficiency with which the facility is conducted, and on the following factors.

1 The turnover of stock. A quick turnover of drugs means that large amounts of capital are not held up for lengthy periods, although inevitably some drugs become obsolete and may have to be discarded. Some dispensing practices are able to control this by means of a stock control computer programme, which allows for re-ordering when stocks reach a certain level.
2 Discounts obtained from pharmaceutical suppliers. The supply of drugs of this nature is highly competitive and there are generally discounts available to practices which can take advantage of them.

On the other hand, partners in a dispensing practice are usually required to contribute a higher level of capital than those in a similar, but non-dispensing, practice. The required stock of drugs, even if kept at a reasonably low level, together with the fact that drug refunds are received up to three months in arrears, means that the current assets of the practice are likely to run at a high level. The high earnings of the partners in part represent a return on this higher investment in the practice capital.

Payments by the FHSA

Drug refunds to dispensing practices are nearly always made in arrears, sometimes by three months, although in the majority of cases payments on account are obtained one or two months in arrears. At any given date, such practices therefore carry a substantial amount of capital. They should try to ensure that payments on account are received regularly and at as high a level as can be negotiated, although the partners must accept that carrying relatively high levels of working capital is one of the obligations of running a dispensing practice.

Superannuation

As we have seen, part of the remuneration of the dispensing GP is in the form of a dispensing fee for each scrip submitted. Such dispensing fees are fully superannuable and are subject to deductions at the standard rate of 6%, or higher if any of the doctors are buying added years.

It is essential that superannuation deductions are identified and shown, as with similar deductions from fees and allowances, as part of the charge to each individual doctor through their own current accounts. The practice should ensure that proper elections are submitted to the FHSA so that these contributions are allocated in partnership ratios.

Stock on hand

At each annual account date, the stock of drugs should be properly valued and shown in the accounts at that value.

Many practices employ specialist valuers who come to the surgery shortly after close of business on an account date, to count and check the drugs on hand. These can, if necessary, be valued first and the calculations made at a later date. The stock on hand should include VAT at the rate in force, which would have been paid on these drugs when they were bought. Some practices prefer to have such valuations taken by the doctors and staff, if necessary paying overtime in respect of the additional work entailed.

The valuation should be made on the basis of cost or market value, whichever is the lower. If drugs have been bought at a specially discounted rate, which was less than their true value, it is this rate which should be taken into account when the drugs are valued. Drugs which have no value, or which have been given free by representatives, should not be included in the valuation.

It is essential that this valuation is made and included in the practice accounts. If, as occasionally occurs, a nominal value is included, or worse, the stock is ignored, the profits of the practice will have been understated and the Inland Revenue would be justified in re-assessing the tax, possibly for several years previously.

Prescribing doctors

GPs in non-dispensing practices can, under SFA Section 44.5, claim a refund and fee under similar arrangements to those outlined above. This normally applies to the supply of vaccines, anaesthetics, injections and family planning devices, etc.

However, if the dispensing practitioner supplies a prescription to a patient, with that patient's consent, rather than supplying the drug from his own dispensary, no remuneration will be paid.

The accounts in Chapter 18 (pages 98–112) are for a dispensing practice. Figure 33.1 calculates profit earned by that practice over two years.

	1993		1992	
	£	£	£	£
Cost of goods sold (*see* page 106)				
Stock at 1 July		3940		3228
Puchases during year		37 761		36 174
		41 701		39 402
Less: stock at 30 June 1993		4275		3940
Cost of drugs dispensed (Note 13)		37 426		35 462
Proceeds:				
Refunds (including VAT, etc) (Note 10)	49 745		38 877	
Dispensing fees (Note 9)	3462	53 207	2546	41 423
Dispensing profit for the year		15 781		5961
Percentage profit return		29.7%		14.4%

The practice has improved its profitability from its dispensing facility, both in terms of actual profit realized and the percentage return. This may have come about through increased efficiency, improved stock control, a higher discount available, or a combination of all three. Where amounts are received by way of private prescriptions, total income from this source should be included in such a trading account.

The figures are taken from the specimen accounts in Chapter 18, pages 98–112.

Figure 33.1   The trading account of a dispensing practice

34 The Fundholding Practice

A facility for GPs to hold their own practice budgets, administering these extensive funds on behalf of the NHS, came into being on 1 April 1991, and some 300 practices registered as 'first wave' fundholders. The scheme has expanded significantly, with a similar number of new entrants on 1 April 1992 and a further 600 on 1 April 1993, as 'third wave' fundholders.

GP fundholding is largely an exercise in finance and management and it is essential that all practices have a high level of knowledge and understanding of these aspects of the scheme. Whilst the clinical aspect is important and indeed the major purpose of the exercise, fundholding also fulfils the Government's aim to control NHS spending, particularly in the field of family practitioner services.

Knowledge of the scheme should be kept up to date as the rules are constantly changing.

Eligibility for fundholding

Whilst entry to the fundholding scheme is voluntary, certain criteria must be satisfied before a practice is allowed to participate.

1 A minimum list size of 7000 patients (from 1 April 1993). However, small practices whose list sizes fall below this level are permitted to join together, sharing a fund between them and administering it jointly. In addition, a few 'development practices' have gone into the scheme with the object of ascertaining the viability of fundholding in small practices.
2 All partners in the practice must participate in the scheme. In practice, it is unlikely to be successful unless all the patners give it a high level of commitment.
3 The practice must be able to demonstrate the standards of efficiency and resources necessary to manage the fund in a manner acceptable to the RHA.
4 The practice must have a fully operational computer system at the commencement of its first fundholding year, by which means the fund can be administered. Fundholding cannot be carried on with a manual system of control.
5 A high level of information on hospital referral rates must be provided to the regional health authority (RHA) during the preparatory year, so that the level of the initial fund can be determined.

Responsibility and control

The RHA, to whom all FHSAs report, carries the ultimate responsibility for the practice fundholding system, and is directly responsible to the Department of Health. The RHA is responsible for determining eligibility, approving practices and setting the level of each fund.

The FHSA is responsible for the day to day monitoring of fundholding and is the authority to which fundholders should submit their monthly accounts and activity reports. The FHSA not only monitors the financial implications of fundholding, reporting to the RHA, but also the quality of services provided to patients in the area.

The FHSA holds the fund on the practice's behalf and is the paying agent for invoices from providers and for prescribing costs from the PPA. Payments are normally made monthly to fundholding practices by the FHSA, either on the basis of cash requisitions or in respect of the budget for staffing costs. The FHSA also pays over to the practice refunds of sums paid out of the management allowance.

Administration of the fund

The initial responsibility for the conduct of the fund at practice level lies with the partners and their fund manager. Although overseen by the FHSA and RHA, the practice has a great deal of autonomy, and fundholding practices must understand the nature of their duties in this respect.

Accounting implications

Originally issued in 1990, and updated during 1993, the GP Fundholder's Manual of Accounts sets down the accounting procedures and detailed entries which are required in the fundholding accounting system.

This system is based upon normal double entry accounting procedures. All accounts, which are made up to 31 March annually for the fundholding facility, are prepared on an accruals basis by which costs are recorded in the periods during which they were incurred, rather than those in which they are paid. The software computer systems available to fundholding practices provide a high level of automatic processing for the accounting entries. This applies particularly to the recording of hospital services.

A high level of accounting knowledge and skill is required in order that the system is operated properly and it is recommended that practices ensure that managers have that standard of knowledge. Alternatively, this must be 'bought in' from a professional accountant specializing in the field.

Virement

Although the budget is presented in three separate components, it is viewed by the health authority as a single fund, so that the practice is not restricted to spending it in the same proportions as those in which it is presented. If, therefore, the practice is able to show a saving in prescribing costs, this may be used during the same year to cover an overspend on hospital referrals. This process is known as 'virement'. It may be extended in certain circumstances to the staffing costs element included in the budget.

Bank accounts

It will be necessary for a new bank account to be opened, normally at the same bank in which the ordinary practice accounts are kept, in order to keep the funds which do not belong to the practice entirely separate.

The majority of the funds passing through this account will be in respect of payments by the FHSA in respect of the staff element of the budget; out of these the practice will pay to the general practice account, at regular intervals, the refund of staff costs to which they are normally entitled. Bank charges incurred on this account should be included with the management allowance (*see* page 207) and an application for refund made accordingly.

Where these funds are kept in an interest bearing account, any interest credited to the account does *not* belong to the practice, but must be credited through the fundholding accounting system back to the FHSA.

Hospital and community health services expenditure

The provider units in this case are paid directly by the FHSA without any cash passing through the practice, although fundholding practices are responsible for the authorization and checking of invoices. A remittance advice is produced (Fund Schedule 9) and sent to the FHSA which then pays the provider unit direct.

Where treatment costs in respect of any individual payment exceed £5000 in a single year, such excess must be reclaimed from the patient's DHA via he FHSA. Such claims should normally be sent to the FHSA monthly (Fund Report 4).

Drugs and appliances

The practice will receive a monthly PACT statement, but again will have no part in settling the funds therein, which are paid directly by the FHSA. Such expenditure is recorded in total through the fundholding accounts.

Management and staffing

It is essential that, before the first fundholding year commences, the practice organizes its staffing levels with a proper system of management and control based upon an agreed management structure. This should recognize the skills and abilities of the individuals involved and avoid unnecessary conflict within the practice, yet be sufficiently flexible that it can adapt when changes are required. Ideally, a management chart should be produced which gives everyone concerned a clear indication of where they fit into the system, to whom they report and to whom they might delegate. Such a chart is an essential feature of any business plan produced for a potential fundholding practice.

Figure 34.1 shows two alternative designs for organization charts for fundholding practices. In chart 1, the partners have delegated responsibility for the fund to a fund partner, who in turn reports to an executive committee and to whom the practice manager is answerable. The latter has responsibility for all the normal functions of the practice. Thus, there are two separate and parallel structures. A fund project manager reports directly to the fund partner and delegates to various operators, without being answerable to the practice manager.

Chart 2, on the other hand, shows a rather different picture, with the partners delegating much of their administration function to an executive partner, who in turn delegates to a practice manager who is in charge of the whole of the administration of the practice, including that of the fund. In this second chart, the practice manager is clearly the key figure, and to a large degree the success of the practice and its fund facility depend on her.

These are not the only possible management structures; others are available and in use. Whichever system suits the practice, however, should be in use by the time fund holding proper commences. It must also be borne

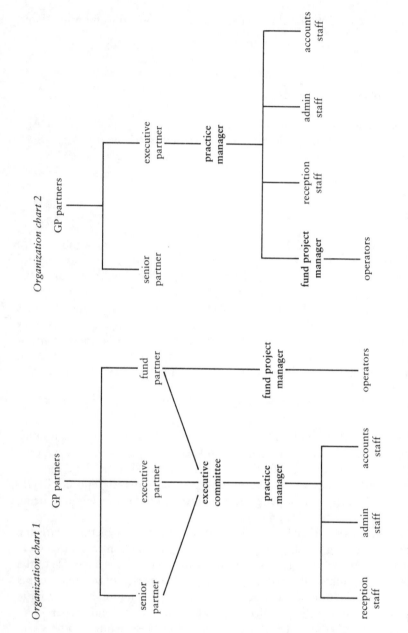

Organization chart 1

GP partners

senior partner — executive partner — fund partner

executive committee

fund partner — fund project manager — operators

practice manager

reception staff — admin staff — accounts staff

Organization chart 2

GP partners

senior partner — executive partner

practice manager

fund project manager — operators

reception staff — admin staff — accounts staff

Figure 34.1 Alternative organization charts for managing a fundholding practice

in mind that even the best management structures can fall down when people are sick or absent, or when staff leave. In such cases, there should ideally be a ready-made substitute who can stand in during such periods of absence or emergency. Certainly, the responsible partner should have a detailed working knowledge of the scheme and be able to step in when all else fails.

The management allowance

A principle of the fundholding scheme is that practices are paid a prescribed maximum sum, out of which they can fund additional expenses incurred in administering their fund. This is known as the management allowance. The upper level of this allowance for the year 1993–4 is £35 000. Half of this (£17 500) is available for practices during their preparatory year, ie the 12 months immediately prior to them entering the scheme proper. This is a maximum figure; if total expenditure falls short of that figure, no additional amount will be paid.

Expenditure which might be included within the management allowance includes such items as staffing, professional fees, business planning, staff training and equipment, as well as incidental costs such as telephone charges, stationery and postage, etc. Up to 50% of the preparatory year allowance may be used to cover the purchase of capital equipment, which for this purpose is defined as items costing £1000 or more. An element of reimbursement is also allowed for locums, and deputizing by partners in the practice, up to a level of £3718. After the practice has become fundholding, the locum allowance cannot be used to pay partners of the practice.

There are also generous additional reimbursements for computer equipment (see Chapter 20), maintenance and support, and the cost of fundholding software maintenance and training is partially reimbursable by the FHSA in addition to the management allowance.

Figure 34.2 sets out how a management allowance might be allocated for both the preparatory and fundholding years.

Business planning

We have seen (Chapter 14) how practices can obtain assistance towards the cost of business planning. In the case of fundholding practices, however, it is not normal to allow a 'double funding', ie part funding for the same plan from the management allowance and from the DTI grant.

	Preparatory year	1st fundholding year
	£	£
Staff salaries	9000	22 000
Training costs	2000	1500
Equipment hire and maintenance	500	1500
Postage and stationery	50	200
Bank charges	50	100
Capital costs: equipment	2500	2000
Professional fees:		
Business planning	1750	–
Accountancy	–	1800
Computer support	1000	3000
Telephone/fax	400	2500
Sundry expenses	250	400
	17 500	35 000

Figure 34.2   Allocation of a fundholding management allowance

Any business plan funded from the management allowance must normally consider only the aspects of the practice relating to the fundholding facility, such as management structures, the roles of the partners and staff, and financing arrangements. It cannot, for instance, look at the overall profitability levels, cash flow and drawings in respect of the practice and the individual partners.

Whilst the preparation of such a business plan is not mandatory, many RHAs have insisted on it as an essential preliminary to practices attaining fundholding status. Many such plans have been prepared by practices themselves and have not addressed the full implications of the steps they are proposing to take. It is strongly recommended that business plans be prepared by outside consultants, who have detailed knowledge of practice finance in general and the fundholding scheme in particular; a rather more detached view can then be taken than would otherwise be possible. The consultant's fee for preparing the plan, and any costs, can be taken out of the management allowance.

Fund savings

Any underspend on the budget during a single year can be retained by the practice to spend on improving the standards of care for their patients. Such expenditure can only be authorized after the accounts have been approved by the auditors and the fund savings confirmed. It is not permitted either to make such expenditure out of fund savings before these are confirmed by the auditors, or to reimburse expenditure retrospectively out of such savings.

Fund savings may only be carried forward for four years before they are cancelled and the remaining savings credited back to the FHSA.

Fundholding and general practice accounts

As we have seen, the fundholding accounts system is entirely separate from the practice accounts. Indeed, it is unlikely that the fundholding accounting year-end on 31 March will correspond to that of the practice. Despite this, there are several aspects of fundholding which do affect the practice accounts, and these should be taken into consideration when accounts are prepared.

1 The fundholding bank account is not the property of the partners and should not appear on the balance sheet of the general practice.
2 Interest and charges on the fundholding account should be debited directly to the general practice account and reimbursement claimed via the management allowance.
3 The management allowance, both for the preparatory and the fundholding years, must be shown as separate items of income and expenditure in order to 'gross up' practice expenditure for Review Body purposes. The reason for this is fully explained in Chapter 3.
4 Where capital equipment has been purchased and reimbursed out of the management allowance, or other grant sources, this should be shown as grants in the fixed asset notes to the accounts in order to reduce the cost of the assets to the practice. In many cases, this net cost will be reduced to nil. Capital allowances for taxation purposes may be claimed only on net cost to the practice.
5 Reimbursements out of the staff fund for the general practice must be included in the practice accounts as ancillary staff refunds, and care must be taken to ensure that all money due to the practice for the year has been included.
6 At any given date, there will be a balance on the general practice account within the fundholding accounts system. It must be ensured that this balance is included in the practice accounts as an item of debt or credit, whichever applies.

Requirements for audit

The Fundholder's Manual of Accounts provides for audits to be carried out by the Audit Commission at three yearly intervals. However, all accounts for first and second wave fundholders are audited after their first year of operation and it is anticipated that this process will continue. It has recently been announced that all first wave fundholders will also have their second year's accounts audited in order to ensure that the recommendations made at the time of the first audit have been implemented.

The Audit Commission also have a right of access to the accounting records of the general practice, and fundholding practices should ensure that these are made available on request. In practice, this power is only exercised in exceptional circumstances.

Chapter 18, page 107, shows a typical fund income and expenditure account extracted from the fundholding accounting system.

Further reading

Fundholding magazine (Haymarket Publications) is sent without charge to all fundholding practices.

Fundholding: a practice guide, Second Edition (Radcliffe Medical Press): £13.50.

Extracts from *The new practice manager* (Radcliffe Medical Press), issued with Practice Manager Development courses.

35 The Single-handed Practitioner

THE majority of GPs in this country practise as members of partnerships. The single-handed practitioner is now in the minority, yet it is a status that retains a few advantages for those who wish to practise in this manner.

Advantages of single-handed practice

The advantages are chiefly related to independence. Some single-handed practitioners have been members of partnerships and either have not relished the experience or find difficulty in working with close colleagues. However, the complexities of modern medical finance and the advantages of forming partnerships are such that the number of single-handed GPs is likely to gradually diminish.

Disadvantages of single-handed practice

Out-of-hours work

Single-handed GPs, particularly in rural areas, find it difficult to obtain assistance with night and other duties. In urban areas, some may join rotas, but for others the use of locums and deputizing services is expensive and is likely to become more so following the introduction of differential rates for payment of night duty fees.

Reference and discussion

Many single-handed GPs find that they are remote from their professional colleagues; they do not have the closeness of the members of a successful partnership, and can at times find it difficult to discuss common problems with their peers.

Earnings levels

The need to cover fully the cost of the various services a GP must use, such as telephone, postage and stationery, and accountancy, may reduce earnings.

The average single-handed GP has none of the benefits of the pooling of expenses which takes place in a partnership.

At times of sickness and holidays he is obliged to use the services of locums, which may not be necessary even in a medium-sized partnership.

24-hour retirement

The single-handed GP who contemplates taking a 24-hour retirement is virtually prohibited from doing so by application of the abatement rule (*see* Chapters 47 and 48). The main benefit of such a partial retirement is the possibility of reducing working hours, which cannot apply to the single-handed GP who can only cover the work he seeks not to do by the engagement of locums or other doctors. If he continues to earn gross fees from the NHS at the pre-retirement rate, his pension is likely to be abated such that the benefits of partial retirement will be negated.

Appointment of a successor

The single-handed GP has no right to appoint a successor, as does a GP in partnership. On retirement, the vacancy will be put up for interview by the local medical commitee and the FHSA, so that he will have no voice in choosing a successor to cater for his patients. Some single-handed GPs seek to counteract this by taking a partner or assistant for a year or two before retirement, but this is subject to approval by the FHSA.

Accounts and finance

In terms of book-keeping, the single-handed practitioner should keep records virtually akin to those kept by a partnership, with the exception of calculating drawings and balancing capital accounts. He will, however, still need to have capital invested in his practice, albeit to a somewhat smaller degree.

The single-handed GP should open a practice bank account, into which all medical earnings are paid and from which will be settled all expenses wholly or partially of a business nature. At the end of the month, he can transfer into his private account such sums as appear reasonable taking into account future known commitments.

If a single-handed GP seeks to develop his own surgery, as some do, he may encounter difficulties in borrowing money due to his non-partnership status.

Single-handed GPs in isolated areas may be able to engage the services of an assistant doctor and receive the associate allowance to partly fund the salary. Such GPs must be in receipt of rural practice payments, or be practising on an island, and either be in receipt of an inducement payment or the practice should be more than 10 miles from the nearest main surgery or district general hospital.

Compliance with legislation

The single-handed GP, who will probably have a very limited staff, is likely to experience difficulty in both keeping up to date and complying with the bureaucracy and all-pervading legislation which is part of the life of any self-employed businessman and employer. Such legislation as the Data Protection Act, Health and Safety Acts, employment legislation, PAYE and National Insurance and planning regulations take up a great deal of time. Many GPs prefer to spend their time dealing with patients, as they were trained to do, yet single-handed GPs are unable to share responsibility for dealing with legislative issues.

36 Women Doctors

IN an increasing number of cases, the woman GP is either the bread winner or the major earner in the family. Female doctors experience many problems in terms of clinical matters and sex discrimination, and also financial and management problems specific to their sex. It is therefore necessary that the woman doctor, particularly one on the point of entering general practice, is aware of these and is able to cater for them as far as possible.

The increasing number of women GPs and the impact that they are having on general practice can be seen from a recent statistic which showed that there were 7137 women GP principals in England and Wales, representing 35% of all GPs. This would suggest a UK total of about 11 500 out of 33 000 GPs. Taking into account the number of young woman doctors currently qualifying, it is evident that the trend will continue to be upwards, and the problems of women GPs are thus likely to magnify over the years.

In conventional society, women not only bear the children but are charged with the responsibility of raising them within the family. It is also normal practice, but by no means universal, in our society that women are the members of the family unit invariably charged with the routine tasks of catering for the family household and ensuring that it runs in as smooth and efficient a manner as possible. Hence the problems and prejudices that affect working women.

Job sharing

One of the more novel aspects of the 1990 GP contract was its introduction of 'job sharing' as a legally recognized option, particularly to cater for the aspirations of female doctors who cannot devote the whole of their lives and working hours to their practice. The detailed conditions for this are set out in Chapter 37.

A further variation of the job sharing facility is the manner in which it has been extended to husband and wife GP teams in a more flexible form. Whilst unrelated job sharers are likely to allocate their minimum 26 hours per week more or less equally, a husband and wife may choose instead for one partner, say the husband, to work twenty hours and his wife six; this is quite acceptable as long as the contract is fulfilled and the practice works in an efficient manner. Such a situation may be compared favourably with the position of other part-time practitioners (*see* Chapter 37) who are required to work at least 13 hours a week in order to qualify for the BPA.

Maternity allowance

A female employee is entitled to certain protection with regard to maternity leave and her job must be kept open during her absence. However, this does not apply to female GPs, who are not employees but independent contractors who are self-employed. They can nevertheless claim certain allowances under the terms of this contract with the NHS.

Detailed conditions for payment of the maternity allowance to female GPs (referred to as additional payments during confinement) are set out in paragraph 49 of the SFA. Generally, the scheme operates on a similar basis to payment during absence through sickness, although there is now no restriction in respect of minimum list sizes.

Payments under the maternity scheme are made to any GP on the medical list, provided she expresses an intention to continue in general practice. They are intended to reimburse her wholly, or partly, for the cost of an external locum whom she has engaged to give clinical care to patients during her absence. Where the doctor in question is a part-time practitioner or job sharer, payments are scaled down accordingly.

Payments will normally continue for a period of 13 weeks maximum, or until such time as the GP re-enters practice. If it is necessary for the practitioner to be away from her practice for longer than 13 weeks due to ill health, she may be able to claim payments under the sickness scheme, although she cannot benefit from both the sickness and maternity schemes simultaneously.

It is essential that the practitioner who either is, or anticipates finding herself, absent from the practice through childbirth, agrees with her partners the exact financial conditions which are to apply and that these are set down in a proper partnership deed. Partnership deeds are considered more fully in Chapter 22 and maternity leave provisions are considered on pages 139–40.

Partnership deeds

It is essential that a female GP, preferably on joining a practice, agrees with her partners the exact financial provisions which are to apply in the event of any future absence on maternity leave.

There are two main variations which can apply, and a choice will be made according to the policy of the partnership.

1 The female GP pays the locums herself during the entire period of her absence and retains the maternity allowance during the 13 week period, or whatever period is covered.
2 All transactions are passed through the partnership, which pays the locum fees and retains the maternity allowance.

Under the first of these options, any shortfall in cost is automatically borne by the absent GP, whilst in the second case any shortfall is covered by the partnership.

For practical reasons, it is better if the locum is physically paid by the female GP out of her own funds and the maternity allowance paid to her on receipt. This avoids confusion where GPs are absent for more than 13 weeks, but the allowance is limited to that length of time. The payment of locums in such circumstances is best kept outside the partnership accounts, as when the accountant comes to draw them up, up to a year later, it may be forgotten which locum fees apply to the maternity period.

Child minding

Female GPs are unable to obtain tax relief for the cost of engaging people to look after their children whilst they are at work. The case is often made that most women GPs would not be able to work without such a facility and that it is a legitimate charge against tax. Unfortunately, such logic is lost on the Inland Revenue, which consistently declines to accept any such claims. In recent years, some relief has been granted where an employer provides a creche or similar facility for the children of its employees, but this is not extended to self-employed GPs or indeed to any other cases where child minding fees are paid in cash by the claimant.

Salaries for husbands

Chapter 43 (page 260) addresses the issue of female doctors paying a salary to their husbands for assistance in their practice. Such a payment is permitted, although it is likely to be less tax efficient than the reverse situation of a husband paying a salary to his wife for assistance in the practice. Page 260 also discusses payments to older children for similar duties.

Wives' pension schemes

These are covered in some detail on page 260. However, in the case of a female GP who is the wife of a male GP, then it is more likely that the claim will be accepted, as the woman's professional qualification obviously gives her a great deal of value in assisting her husband.

In such circumstances, and particularly if the woman GP has no other source of income, it is essential that the husband pays employee pension premiums on her salary. This, it is suggested, should be an investment priority for the family.

Widowers' pensions

Since 6 April 1988, contributions made by female GPs to the NHS Pension Scheme (NHSPS) have also contributed to the purchase of a pension for the widower in the event of the woman's death either during service or in retirement. Until 30 June 1989, it was possible for female GPs to buy benefit arrears, but this is no longer available and any contributions made will only count towards a widower's pension from 1988. Female doctors who feel that they have not made adequate pension provision should consider the various private pension schemes which are now available. (*See* Chapters 47 and 48.)

Surgery ownership

Many female GPs, on entering a practice, do not take part in the acquisition of a share in the surgery building, possibly due to the uncertain duration of their stake in the partnership; for example, they may at some time be required to move location as a result of their husband's employment, or for another reason.

This decision can only be made by the practitioner concerned, in consultation with her partners. However, despite recent problems with negative equity (*see* Chapter 29), ownership of surgeries is an excellent long-term investment, and GPs who decline the opportunity to take part in ownership may well be losing, not only a valuable continuing source of income, but also a significant tax-free capital sum on retirement. Women GPs who anticipate remaining with the practice for a lengthy period should seriously consider buying into the surgery.

Where the GP does not take on the responsibility of surgery ownership, and will not share in any proceeds of the cost or notional rent reimbursement, she should ensure that she is not required to pay any share of interest or repayments on the surgery mortgage, or to pay rent to her partners for the privilege of practising from the surgery.

37 Part-time Working

Position prior to April 1990

HITHERTO, the nature of the GP contract and its associated remuneration structure made the concept of a part-time GP all but irrelevant. Within a partnership, the commitment of an individual partner, whether set out in relation to duties or hours, was a matter for agreement, as were the relative rewards to the partners. The only implications of what might, in other walks of life, be deemed part-time working were restricted to whether the practitioner concerned could satisfy the criteria for receipt of the full rate of allowances (principally the BPA) and be deemed a true partner in accordance with the regulations. These criteria were a personal list of 1000 patients or an average list of 1000 within a partnership and devotion of a substantial amount of time to general practice.

The SFA indicated that the second of these criteria would normally be met where services to patients were given by the GP concerned, whether in surgery or in the home, on average over the year during 20 hours per week at times reasonably spread over the normal week. These criteria were quite permissive and general practice partnerships were able to absorb a variety of commitments at no loss of aggregate income to the partnership, whilst maintaining equity of treatment to individual partners. In order to be satisfied that the practitioner with a limited commitment to the partnership was truly a partner, the FPC had regard to the regulation whereby a practitioner had to receive a share of the partnership profits at least equal to one-third of the share of the partner with the largest share.

Arrangements from 1 April 1990

Under the new contractual arrangements and revised regulations, arrangements were introduced to formalize, for the first time, part-time working in general practice. These arrangements were foreshadowed in the White Paper, *Promoting Better Health*, published in November 1987 and were originally designed to encourage more women to enter and remain in general practice. They are not, however, restricted to women doctors. The new arrangements provide for the formal status of job sharer and part-time practitioner.

Job sharers

Until April 1990, job sharing did not formally exist within general practice, although it is believed that a substantial number of informal arrangements operated with tacit approval. Essentially, job sharers are now treated jointly as a single practitioner and thus they are jointly eligible for a single BPA. The amended regulations set out how such GPs will satisfy the availability provisions. Each GP will normally be available for less than 26 hours in a week, but they will in aggregate be available for no less than 26 hours in any such week. The essential difference between a job sharer and a part-time practitioner is eligibility for the BPA and the additions to it. Job sharers, by being jointly eligible for a single BPA, have this calculated in accordance with their aggregate list size (average list size in a partnership) and their personal list sizes are disregarded.

From the financial point of view, partnerships considering job sharing arrangements for partners will need to bear in mind that, whilst for most purposes the two job sharers can be regarded as a single entity, there will be some expenses which, when taken jointly, will be greater than those incurred for a single partner.

Part-time practitioners

This option is only open to members of a partnership where at least one partner is a full-time practitioner. The part-time practitioner is eligible for one BPA, the level of which is determined by a notional list of patients, which in turn is dictated by the hours of availability under the terms of service. Thus, a GP who is normally available for less than 26 hours but not less than 19 hours each week, for 42 weeks of the year, will be deemed a three-quarter practitioner, and the amount of BPA to which he is entitled will be no greater than that payable for a list of 900 patients. Similarly, a GP available for less than 19 hours per week, but not less than 13 hours, will be deemed a half-time practitioner and will be eligible for a BPA no greater than that payable in respect of 600 patients. If the practitioner's personal or average partnership list is smaller than the appropriate limit then that list will dictate the amount of BPA; if the list is greater, the notional list size will apply.

Consequently, there has been an amendment to the regulations dealing with status as a partner. In short, the one-third rule has been amended so that, for a three-quarter time practitioner, the relevant share of the profits is now not less than one-quarter of the share of the partner with the greatest share, and for a half-time practitioner it is one-fifth.

The status of part-timer relates solely to considerations of availability for surgery consultations, clinics and visits. In all other respects, the GP's obligations are no different to those of a full-time practitioner.

The method of calculating partnership average list size, and thus eligibility for levels of BPA in practices with part-time practitioners, has been set to minimize the need for moving patients between personal lists to maximize income. The two examples below show the manner of the calculation.

Example 1
  A: Full-time partner with list of 1000 patients.
  B: Full-time partner with list of 1300 patients.
  C: Half-time practitioner with list of 700 patients.

For purposes of calculating BPA entitlement, the aggregate list is divided by 2.5 and this becomes the list for the full-time partners. Thus, notional lists are:

  A: 1200
  B: 1200
  C: 600

Example 2
  A: Full-time partner with list of 1500 patients.
  B: Three-quarter practitioner with list of 700 patients.
  C: Full-time partner with list of 1200 patients.

For purposes of calculating BPA entitlement, the aggregate list is divided by 2.75 and this becomes the list for the full-time partners. Thus, notional lists become:

  A: 1236
  B: 927
  C: 1236

Figures now available show that the total numbers of GPs in England and Wales in October 1992 were divided as follows:

Full-time	25 333
Job share	483
Half-time	621
Quarter-time	1207
Total	27 644

38 Taxation in General Practice

'For God's sake madam, don't say that in England, for if you do, they will surely tax it.'

Jonathan Swift

TAXATION of some kind has always been with us and presumably will remain. It comes in several forms: taxes on income, on capital, on the estates of deceased persons and value added tax levied on goods and services. A GP is likely to come across most, if not all, of those forms of taxation during his working life.

The purpose of this chapter is to explain, particularly to new GPs, the principles that apply and the manner in which income from their practices is taxed. Taxation of all types is extremely complex and GPs are well advised to engage the services of a qualified, experienced and specialist accountant to give advice on all aspects of tax. Once an accountant has been employed, the GP should *not* negotiate and correspond separately with the local tax office.

The regulation of taxes is based upon Acts of Parliament which lay down, in general terms, the means by which those taxes are to be levied, administered and collected. Each year, from 1993 in November, the Chancellor of the Exchequer presents to Parliament a Budget Statement, which ultimately becomes the Finance Act for that year. From time to time the various regulations and statutes are codified in an omnibus act, the latest of these being the Income and Corporation Taxes Act, 1988.

The Inland Revenue offices

As far as the GP is concerned, the Revenue service is divided into two sections: the Inspector and the Collector. It is the Inspector of Taxes office with which an accountant negotiates in order to agree a client's tax liability. The office is staffed by revenue officials of various grades who each have their separate function to perform. It is that office which issues assessment notices, to which appeals will be sent and with which correspondence is conducted.

The Collector of Taxes offices throughout the country are responsible for the demand and collection of tax. It is this office to which a tax bill is paid, and which deals with the issue of receipts and takes enforcement proceedings if the tax is not paid.

The various schedules

Income tax is divided into several schedules, each of which governs the rules for assessment of tax on incomes of various types. The schedules currently in force are set out in Box 38.1.

Box 38.1: Income tax: the various schedules

Schedule A: Income from property
Schedule B: Woodlands
Schedule C: Paying agents
Schedule D: Cases I and II: Profits from trades, professions, etc
              Case III: Interest receivable
              Cases IV and V: Overseas income
              Case VI: Miscellaneous income
Schedule E: Earnings from employment: salaries, wages, etc
Schedule F: Dividends, etc.

Employment and self-employment: Schedules D and E

For most GPs, the tax upon their incomes will be of greatest concern, and Schedules D and E will be most relevant. The main characteristics of each schedule are set out in Box 38.2.

Box 38.2: Income tax: Schedules D and E

Schedule D
- Paid by self-employed (including GPs).
- Assessed on preceding year basis.
- Payable in arrears, usually twice a year.
- More relaxed treatment of expense claims (but *see* Chapter 41 on the detailed preparation of these claims).
- National Insurance: classes 2 and 4 (*see* Chapter 44).

Box 38.2: *continued*

Schedule E

- Paid by employees (practice staff, GP trainees, hospital doctors, etc).
- Assessed on actual year basis, and paid over monthly.
- Payable by deduction from wages/salaries. Stringent treatment of claims for expenses.
- National Insurance: class 1 (*see* Chapter 44).

Most GPs at some time will have been assessed for tax under Schedule E and have had deductions made from their salaries under PAYE; they may have been employees of a hospital authority, GP trainees or in other forms of employment.

The GP as a self-employed practitioner is assessed under Schedule D, which derives entirely from his status as an independent contractor.

As the method of assessment in each schedule is different, it is important to understand how these schedules work. The main differences lie in the manner in which expenses are allowed, the basis of assessment, and the dates of payment of tax. These rules apply to *all* self-employed taxpayers. The taxation problems arising in medical partnerships are discussed more fully in Chapter 39, whilst personal expenses claims are dealt with in Chapter 41.

In many cases, these two schedules overlap, with some GPs receiving income simultaneously under both headings. Where this occurs in partnerships, extremely complex situations can arise, and these are discussed more fully in Chapter 39.

Moreover, in many cases, it is not immediately apparent whether the income from any particular appointment is to be assessed under Schedule D or Schedule E. In recent years, the Inland Revenue have examined several professions outside the medical world and re-designated them as Schedule E from Schedule D.

In the medical field, confusion can frequently arise in the treatment of fees paid to locums or assistant GPs. Where fees are paid from practice funds, the proper taxation formalities should be observed. For instance, if a practice engages a doctor at a salary of £15 000 a year and then proceeds to pay that doctor monthly, this constitutes a salary and must be taxed under PAYE. On the other hand, if occasional locum fees are paid to different doctors, calculated on a sessional basis without any true employer–employee relationship, then it is likely that they can be treated as Schedule D income and the recipient must bear the obligation of returning these to the Inland Revenue and paying tax upon them.

Years of assessment

Tax is organized on a basis of tax years, sometimes termed 'years of assessment' or 'fiscal years'. In all cases, these years run from 6 April in one calendar year to 5 April in the next. Thus, the year from 6 April 1992 to 5 April 1993 would be designated 1992/93, and that from 6 April 1993 to 5 April 1994 as 1993/94. (*See also* Chapter 21.)

The basis of assessment

A major benefit from Schedule D status is the facility for paying tax in arrears, up to two years after the income was earned. This situation arises from the preceding year basis of assessment, whereas profits charged to tax in any year of assessment are based upon the profits earned in the accounting period ending within the preceding tax year.

Bearing in mind that all tax years run from 6 April in one year to 5 April in the next year, if a practice has its accounts made up to 30 June 1993, the profits would be assessed in the tax year 1994/95. It is interesting to note that if those profits were made up for the year to 31 March 1993, they would be assessed to tax a year earlier, in the 1993/94 year. This gives an opportunity for tax planning in any business and offers the chance of deferring tax for long periods. For instance, in the example already given, profits earned during the 12 months ending 30 June 1993 would not be assessed for tax until the tax year 1994/95, and the tax would be paid some two years after it was earned.

Proposed change in basis of assessment

This preceding year basis of assessment, which is largely beneficial to all self-employed taxpayers, including GPs, is scheduled to change shortly, probably during the 1996/97 tax year, to an actual year basis of assessment. Whilst there will be transitional arrangements to ensure that no-one suffers unduly from the change, on a long-term basis it will mean that GPs will be paying tax on the year's profits somewhat earlier than previously. If one assumes a regime of gradually increasing profits, this will have an adverse effect on the cash flow position of the practice. GPs should therefore discuss with their professional advisers the likely effect of the new basis of assessment on their practices.

Dates of payment of tax

The rule for payment of Schedule D tax to the Inland Revenue is that it is payable in two equal instalments on 1 January during the year of assessment and on 1 July immediately following. Therefore, to take the example quoted above, tax on the profits of the year to 30 June 1993 would be assessed in the year 1994/95 and paid in January and July 1995. To this would be added the Class 4 National Insurance liability (*see* Chapter 44).

Interest is payable on unpaid tax at the rate currently in force, and usually starts to run from the proper due date of payment. If an individual overpays his tax and a repayment is due from the Revenue, this will ultimately be repaid, but interest on this (known as a repayment supplement) will not start to run until one year after the end of the year of assessment concerned.

39 Partnership Taxation

WE have had a look (Chapter 21) at how partnerships in general practice work and have seen how the majority of GPs function as members of partnerships, working together with a view to earning profits and dividing these in agreed ratios. We have also had a look (Chapter 38) at the taxation system in general practice and will see (Chapter 40) how this is applied to individuals.

The majority of GPs are taxed as members of their partnerships. We shall now look at exactly how partnership taxation works; at the manner in which profits are assessed and allocated between partners.

As we have seen, GPs are assessable for tax under Schedule D, by which in a normal year they will pay tax on profits earned in an accounting year ending within the preceding tax year. Exactly the same rules apply to partnerships; where they differ from doctors practising on their own is that a fair and equitable method must be found for allocating, for taxation purposes, the profits earned by the partnership amongst the doctors who are members of that practice.

The rule which applies to all partnerships, both inside and outside the medical world, is basic and and not unduly complex. Shares of profits as agreed by the Inland Revenue are allocated for tax purposes only between the partners on the basis of the profit-sharing ratios within the year of assessment; not within the accounting period for which those profits are calculated. To take an example: Drs A, B, C and D are practising together in partnership. They make up their accounts to 30 June annually. During the year ended 30 June 1992 the partnership has realized a profit of £120 000. If the four are equal partners, they will therefore have earned £30 000 each during that period. However, the tax will not be assessed on that year but, in effect, on the tax year 1993/94. It is the basis upon which profits are shared during the period between 6 April 1993 and 5 April 1994 that is relevant for the purpose of allocating profits for that tax year. Let us say, therefore, that on 1 April 1993, they recruited an additional partner, Dr E, at an initial share of the profits of 10%, with the other four partners each receiving 22.5%. For the 1993/94 year they would in effect be taxed by reference to those ratios, with Dr E being charged tax on £12 000 and the other four partners on £27 000 each, notwithstanding the fact that those profits were earned prior to Dr E joining the partnership.

This rule, enshrined in law, which applies in all cases of assessments on partnership tax, gives rise to certain anomalies but must nevertheless be understood by the GP in practice, and particularly the new partner to whom both Schedule D and partnership taxation will come as a novel experience, probably after spending the whole of his career to date as a salaried employee.

One of the first financial decisions a new partner is likely to be asked to make on joining the practice is whether he should join with his colleagues in signing a continuation election.

Cessation and continuation basis

Few aspects of partnership taxation are so frequently misunderstood as those applying to the situation which arises from a change in a partnership. A change in this sense is a change in the physical constitution of a partnership, ie Dr A leaving or Dr E joining. It does not apply to a change which does not involve outgoing or incoming partners, such as a change in profit-sharing ratios.

Where such a change in partnership occurs, the law says that a business— in this case a medical practice—is deemed to have ceased for tax purposes on the last day of the old partnership, and a new one commenced on the first day of the new practice. For the last three years of the old practice and the first four years of the new partnership, all is assessed on an actual year basis, which is to say that the partnership for that whole period loses the benefit of the preceding year basis of assessment. Needless to say, this is not an acceptable option in most cases; the majority of medical practices' income increases at a fairly steady rate and the preceding year basis would normally be highly beneficial. In most GP partnership changes, it would be little short of a financial disaster were this cessation basis to be imposed.

Fortunately however, there is a way around this, by completing and submitting to the Inland Revenue a form of continuation election. This is a notice, set out on a sheet of paper and signed by all the partners both before and after the date of change, which elects for the assessment of the partnership to be taken on a continuation basis. A typical form of such an election is set out in Figure 39.1, although various forms of wording may be used.

If this election is made, the assessment on the partnership will continue to be made on the same basis as if there had been no change. The principle must, however, follow that those assessments are to be allocated between the partners on the basis of the ratios in force during the year of assessment.

Drs Black, White, Green, Pink & Brown

We, being all the partners both before and after the partnership change on 1 April 1991, hereby elect that, under the provisions of Section 113 Income and Corporation Taxes Act 1988, assessments on the partnership for 1991/92 and succeeding years be made on a continuing basis.

....

Dr W J Black   Dr S C White

....

Dr D M Green   Dr L F Pink

....

Dr R B D Brown

Figure 39.1   Notice of continuation election

Figure 39.2 sets out a fairly simple example of a partnership making up its accounts to 31 March annually, where profits have risen at a fairly steady rate over a seven-year period between 1988/89 and 1991/92. There was a change in partnership on 31 March/1 April 1991.

It will be seen from this that the profits over this period charged on the cessation basis would be £861 000, whereas on the continuation basis they would be £805 000. There is therefore a clear advantage in opting for the continuation basis.

All situations are not as clear cut and where a great advantage is not immediately obvious, it may be necessary for detailed comparisons and tax calculations to be made by the accountant before the election is made or confirmed.

Such an election must be submitted to the Inland Revenue within two years of the date of change, so that in Figure 39.2 the election would have to be submitted by 31 March 1993. If an election is made and it emerges that it would no longer be beneficial, it can be revoked within the same two-year period.

It is usual to give both incoming and retiring partners an indemnity which will protect them against any loss they might occur through signing such an election. A situation can quite easily arise where the effect of the election is

Partnership profits for the year ended 31 March:

	£
1987	110 000
1988	120 000
1989	130 000
1990	138 000
1991	147 000
1992	160 000
1993	166 000

Assessable for tax as follows:

	On cessation basis £	On continuation basis £
1987/88	120 000	110 000
1988/89	130 000	120 000
1989/90	138 000	130 000
1990/91	147 000	138 000
1991/92	160 000	147 000
1992/93	166 000	160 000
	861 000	805 000

Figure 39.2   The continuation election: partnership change 30 March 1990

beneficial to the partnership as a whole, but may be detrimental to one partner. A typical example might be the case of a retiring partner who, in his final year of practice, had incurred extremely large expenses which would normally have been included in a personal expenses claim (*see* Chapter 41) and allowed against his share of the partnership assessment. That doctor would receive no relief for the expenses he has incurred as they would in effect be allowed against the overall partnership assessment after he had retired. In such a case it may be beneficial for him to invoke an indemnity clause, if one is included in his partnership deed.

It must be emphasized that such an indemnity clause, if invoked, must apply to all the years involved and not only to one year in isolation. The indemnity clause should be invoked only if it can clearly be shown that, over the whole of the preceding three year period, a retiring partner would have benefited more by the cessation basis than the continuation basis.

Joint and several liability

The assessments to income tax raised on these partnership profits will not be charged to any individual partner; rather, they will be assessed by way of a form of assessment notice in the name of the partnership. All the partners are therefore liable for the tax on the whole of their partnership profits, after giving effect to such personal expenses and allowances as each partner is able to claim.

Under the principle of joint and several liability, however, the partnership as a whole can be liable to pay the share of the partnership assessment appropriate to a partner who has left the practice.

Let us say, for instance, that partner E leaves the practice on 30 September 1993. He has been in dispute with his partners and they agree that he is to relinquish his partnership. He then disappears; they cannot locate him and find to their horror that when the tax for the 1993/94 year falls payable on 1 January and 1 July 1994, they are liable to pay his share. As he has been in the partnership for half of that tax year, there will be a liability to income tax on him as a partner.

There is in fact a way around this. Funds can be set aside in a separate income tax reserve account or by including a reserve within the accounts so that a partner cannot withdraw funds which will ultimately be needed for settlement of a future tax liability.

Personal practice expenses

The manner in which doctors are able to claim expenses incurred privately against their own share of the partnership income tax assessment is discussed more fully in Chapter 41. Each partner will submit, or have prepared for him by his accountant, an annual claim for personal practice expenses which is allowable against tax in exactly the same manner as partnership profits are assessed, ie on the preceding year basis.

Therefore, if five GPs are in a partnership making up its annual accounts to 30 June, each of them will prepare a practice expenses claim made up to 30 June annually. GPs are not employees and should not prepare expenses claims up to a 5 April year-end unless this happens to coincide with the annual accounting date of the partnership.

These expenses, once formulated and agreed with the Inland Revenue, will be allowed for tax against that partner's share of the profits and no other. In large partnerships these expenses claims can vary widely as partners' personal circumstances may differ considerably. This will inevitably affect their own share of the partnership tax liability.

A problem could arise where a partner retires, and in his last year has incurred expenses which can be claimed against the partnership tax assessment. If, for instance, partner A retired on 31 March 1993 having incurred expenses amounting to £8 000 during the year ending on that date, those expenses, assuming that a continuation election is beneficial, will be allowed against the partnership tax assessment before the year 1993/94. Doctor A, however, will not be there during that year as his partnership has ceased, but those expenses are nevertheless a correct deduction in calculating the partnership tax assessment. The problem is not whether they are deductible, but the manner in which they are to be allowed against each partner.

Although no hard and fast rules can be laid down, it is usual in these circumstances to add such expenses to those of the continuing partners who were in the practice at the date of Dr A's retirement.

The opposite problem occurs where a new partner joins the practice. Let us say that Dr E joins the practice on 1 April 1993. As we have seen, he will have a share of the partnership tax assessment for 1993/94, even though this is based on profits earned during a previous year. However, he will have incurred no practice expenses during that basis period and it is normal in such circumstances to allow him a notional amount against his assessable profits, in this case for 1993/94.

In these circumstances one usually finds that the Inland Revenue do not query the allocation of expenses of this nature, provided that a logical reason can be given for it and, more importantly, that the quantum of the assessment is unchanged.

Seniority awards, etc

These items of income can cause a similar problem, for the same reason. One will usually find that a retiring partner has attracted the top rate of seniority which, in the case of most partnerships, will be allocated to him only and not pooled with partnership profits for assessment. In the case of Dr A, retiring on 31 March 1993, he will have received seniority for that year amounting to £4500, but will not be in the partnership when that income is assessed, during the 1993/94 year. It is normal practice for this to be added to the general pool of partnership profits for division between the partners who are in the practice during the same year.

Interest received

Some partnerships will receive interest on deposit accounts or funds held in building societies and this will normally be paid after the deduction of tax.

This income is not assessable with the remainder of the Schedule D trading profits of the partnership, but will be taken out outside that assessment and will be charged individually to the partners in the proportions in which they have received it. It is usual for those amounts to be entered separately in the personal tax returns of each partner.

The property owning partnership

We have seen in Chapter 27 the manner in which surgery premises are held in partnerships and that these shares of ownership frequently differ from those in which practice profits are shared.

It is necessary in such circumstances to exclude transactions applying to the surgery ownership from the initial allocation for tax purposes, bringing them in at a later stage but dividing the net profit or loss accruing in the shares in which the building is owned during the year of assessment.

Exactly how these adjustments are made in the case of partnership changes is shown in Figure 39.3.

Schedule E remuneration in partnerships

A major problem can arise when a partnership receives income from outside appointments, often with local hospitals, but also with local authorities, public bodies, etc, from which PAYE tax is deducted at source.

We have seen in Chapter 38 how the various schedules of tax apply to different headings of income and it is common in medical practices for GPs to receive income simultaneously, which is properly taxed both under Schedule D and Schedule E. In the case of single-handed practitioners, this presents no undue problems; both headings of income are assessable fully on the doctor himself and, so long as the accountant ensures that his personal allowances are properly granted, it is highly unlikely that he will pay more than his proper tax liability.

In partnerships, however, the situation is much more complex. A typical situation would be one in which five doctors (A, B, C, D and E) practise together, and doctors B and D have appointments at local hospitals which bring in salaries of £4500 and £1500 respectively. This income, however, is not in equity the income of those doctors but, by virtue of their agreement, is aggregable with partnership profits for division in agreed ratios. Indeed, in the unlikely event of those two doctors not paying their salaries into the partnership account, they could be sued for the money.

The problem arises chiefly with the Inland Revenue, which is frequently not prepared to take a more practical approach, but will stick to the letter of the law and regard those two doctors as 'office-holders', insisting on assessing only those doctors to tax on the full amount of their salaries. This gives rise to huge anomalies within the partnership, with those two doctors only being charged with the tax on their salaries. If no adjustment is made, it is obvious that inequity will result, with the other three partners in effect paying no tax on income which is properly theirs. How then can this problem be resolved?

The short answer is that it can be, and frequently is, resolved quite easily, given a co-operative Inspector of Taxes who is prepared to take a realistic attitude. The problem is not so much the amount of tax payable, which is readily and easily quantified, but rather the manner and fairness with which it is distributed between the partners.

By far the most preferred method of doing this is for an 'NT' coding to be given to the source of income concerned (the hospital salary) which will ensure that no PAYE tax is deducted. This then means that the income will be included with the rest of the partnership's profits for assessment under Schedule D; it will be divided between the partners as outlined above and each partner will pay his or her correct share of the tax. Unfortunately, this is not applied universally and in many cases the local Inspector of Taxes will insist on the salary being taxed in the name of the partner by whom the appointment is held. This becomes even less justified when, as frequently occurs, the actual work has been done not only by that partner but also by some of his colleagues.

In this case, there is no option left but to accept the Inspector's decision and to try and maintain fairness by adjusting the partnership Schedule D computation accordingly. How this can be done is set out in Figure 39.3. It will be seen that only Drs B and D hold appointments which will first be added to the partnership profits for the year of assessment and then deducted from the shares of profit applicable to those two partners. This does give some equity between the partners but is by no means perfect. For instance, with Schedule E tax being assessed on an actual year basis, it is necessary to adjust the Schedule D assessment retrospectively after the end of the tax year concerned.

This is an extremely time-consuming procedure and may be quite unnecessarily expensive to the partnership in terms of accounting fees.

Figure 39.3 is a fairly typical example of a partnership income tax computation on a partnership change and demonstrates the correct treatment of:

- Dr A's retirement with transfer of seniority award
- transfer of closing personal practice expenses
- transfer of notional practice expenses to incoming partner (Dr F)
- surgery income (shared only by Drs B, C, D and E)
- adjustment of estimated Schedule E remuneration.

Further reading

For further and more detailed information about partnership taxation, the reader is referred to the successive annual issues of *Tolley's tax planning*, by the same author, which includes a detailed chapter on various aspects of partnership taxation for GPs.

	Total £	Total £	Dr A £	Dr B £	Dr C £	Dr D £	Dr E £	Dr F £
Partnership profit for the year (to 30 June 1992)		152 000						
Add: Dr A's seniority award		4 500						
		156 500						
Less: Assessed Schedule E (actual)	5500							
Surgery income	12 000	17 500						
		139 000						
Profits as adjusted	139 000							
Add: Assessable Schedule E 1993/94 (est)	6000							
	145 000							
Allocated as follows:								
Period to 30 September 1993 (178 days): 23% : 23% : 23% : 23% : 19% : 12% :	70 712			16 264	16 264	16 264	13 435	8485
Period 1 October 1993 to 5 April 1994 (187days): 22% : 22% : 22% : 22% : 22% : 12%	74 288			16 344	16 344	16 344	16 344	8912
	145 000			32 608	32 608	32 608	29 779	17 397
Less: Assessable Schedule E 1993/94 (est)	6000			4500	—	1500	—	—
				28 108	32 608	31 108	29 779	17 397
Seniority awards		5250		2000	2000	1250	—	—
Surgery income		12 000		3000	3000	3000	3000	—
		156 250		33 108	37 608	35 358	32 779	17 397
Less: Personal practice expenses								
As negotiated		23 824	6000	5864	2486	3947	5527	—
Adjust: For Dr A's expenses			(6000)	1500	1500	1500	1500	—
To give Dr F part year's claim				(400)	(400)	(400)	(400)	(1600)
				6964	3586	5047	6627	1600
		132 426		26 144	34 022	30 311	26 152	15 797

(The effect of capital allowances is ignored in this illustration.)

Figure 39.3 Drs A, B, C, D, E and F: Income tax computation and allocation of adjusted profits for the year of assessment 1993/94

40 Personal Taxation

In a publication of this nature, only the most basic of tax rules can be considered. GPs who seek wider knowledge of tax laws as they affect individual tax-payers, should undertake more extensive reading. However, most GPs engage an accountant (*see* Chapter 49) to deal with taxes for them.

Personal allowance

Independent taxation for spouses has affected the manner in which personal allowances are granted, but the situation in which a husband receives a standard personal allowance, with an additional married couple's allowance where both spouses are working, continues. Certain taxpayers above the age of 65 years will be able to claim higher relief, subject to a maximum income limit, and there are additional reliefs for single parent families and some widows.

There is no longer any specific tax relief for dependent children although single-parent families may claim an additional personal allowance.

Appendix B sets out the main personal allowances in force for the 1993/94 year.

Income tax rates

For some years the basic rate of tax has been at 25%, with only one higher rate of tax at 40%. In addition, a lower rate has now been introduced, which for the 1993/94 year will be 20% up to £2500 per annum.

As we shall see in Chapter 47, it is necessary for tax relief on standard superannuation contributions to be claimed and a GP should check that he is in fact receiving such relief. Some GPs choose to opt out of this relief and instead claim much higher relief on private pension contributions. Steps should be taken to ensure that this relief is granted through the income tax assessment of the GP concerned.

Payment of tax

The GP, whether in single-handed practice or in partnership, would normally expect to pay his tax in two equal instalments, on 1 January and 1 July in and immediately following the year of assessment (*see* Chapter 38). In most cases, these payments will in effect be payments on account, as accurate as is possible at that stage, although inevitably after the end of each year there is normally a 'balancing-up' process, in which account is taken of the more accurate information then available about such reliefs as super-annuation, mortgage interest, etc. These details are not always available when the tax payment takes place, which is why many GPs will be subject to small arrears of tax or, in some cases, repayments.

Mortgage interest relief

GPs with private mortgages on their own houses will be able to claim tax relief on the interest charge, but only up to a ceiling of £30 000. Since 1991 this mortgage interest relief has been limited to the basic rate of 25%, which will be reduced to 20% from 1994/95. Interest on mortgages above that level does not normally qualify for relief, although in some cases where GPs can prove that they use their homes for practice purposes, it might be possible to negotiate additional relief.

The MIRAS (Mortgage Interest Relief at Source) system means that such relief is invariably granted at the time the payment is made, by deduction from the interest payment to the bank or building society, and has no effect on the overall tax assessment of the doctor concerned.

Let us then go on to look at the details of the tax liability for a typical GP for the 1993/94 year, which is calculated in Figure 40.1. In this example, Dr C is a member of a partnership which makes up its accounts to 30 September annually. For the year 1993/94 his share of partnership profits, after deduction of practice expenses and capital allowances, is £34 022. He has a non-working wife and claims the full married personal allowance. He is buying added years of superannuation and also has an annual private fee retainer of £1800 which is taken into consideration in calculating his taxable income.

In this illustration, the GP is taxed at a top rate of 40%. If he has any other taxable income from sources outside the practice, this will also be taxable at 40%.

However, although he is paying 40% on the top slice of his income, together with Class 4 National Insurance at 6.3% on part of this, the various claims, allowances and reliefs which he can justify reduce his total tax and NIC liability to £8264, which is only 21% of his total gross income of £39 408 (£37 608* + £1800).

This illustration takes no account of tax relief on mortgage interest, which would be deducted at source at the basic rate.

	£	£
Dr C: Share of partnership profits (per computation:, see Figure 39.3, page 236)		34 022
Less: Superannuation (including added years)	2750	
Class 4 NIC relief (*see* Chapter 44)	488	
Personal allowance	3445	
Married couple's allowance	1720	
	8403	
Less: Private fee income	1800	
		6603
Taxable income		27 419
Tax calculated as follows:		
2500 @ 25%		500.00
21 200 @ 25%		5300.00
3719 @ 40%		1487.60
27 419		7287.60
Class 4 NIC (maximum)		976.50
Total liability		8264.10

Figure 40.1 Tax liability for a typical GP in 1993/94

---

*See Figure 39.3.

41 Personal Expenses Claims

THERE are few areas that cause such controversy as the extent and manner in which the GP claims tax relief in respect of expenses paid privately, but which wholly or partly involve practice use. It is an area likely to bring the GP into dispute with his accountant and, possibly, the Inland Revenue.

The attitude of the Inland Revenue has changed considerably in recent years; over-claiming of personal expenses by GPs can have serious consequences.

Partnership or personal expenses?

Most of the expenditure met by a GP or, more likely, his partnership, is not likely to be disputed by the Inland Revenue, eg printing and stationery, surgery telephone bills, staff wages and locum fees.

The categories of expenditure paid personally vary from one partnership to another. The policy of the partners will determine what expenditure is paid out of partnership funds and what is paid privately. Whatever the policy, it should be mutually agreed and set down in the partnership deed. It is important for an incoming partner to determine exactly which expenses have to be met personally.

The major items of expenditure likely to be paid personally by the partners are set out in Box 41.1. Of these, spouses' salaries (*see* Chapter 43) and motor expenses (Chapter 42) are dealt with later.

Box 41.1: Practice expenses: Items likely to be paid personally

- House expenses.
- Motor expenses.
- Spouse's salary, pension, etc.
- Defence society and other medical subscriptions.
- Private telephone bills.
- Personal locum fees.

The basic rule

The basic rule applicable to the claiming of personal expenses, for Schedule D purposes, is that they must be seen by the Inland Revenue as having been expended wholly and exclusively for the purpose of the profession.

Thus, the GP who pays locum fees to another doctor for covering his out-of-hours duties, is allowed those fees for income tax purposes. If he were an employed doctor, it is highly unlikely that the expense would be allowed because the additional qualifying word in the case of Schedule E expenses, 'necessarily', might be impossible to justify.

Claims for personal practice expenses in respect of GPs in partnership should always be made up to the same date as the practice's accounting year-end, even if a GP joined mid-way through the year. Thus, if Dr E joined the partnership on 1 February 1993 and the partnership makes up its accounts to 30 June annually, Dr E's first claim should be for the five-month period to 30 June 1993, and to that same annual date in succeeding years.

Of far greater difficulty are those expenses which the GP pays partially for private and partially for practice use—for instance, a private car or telephone used for practice purposes. In fractional terms, the appropriate amount to claim may be the subject of negotiations between the accountant and the Inland Revenue.

A further concept the Inland Revenue applies is 'duality of purpose'. What this means is that if expenditure is incurred simultaneously both for private and practice use, the expenditure will be wholly disallowable. This is subject to a number of interpretations, most of which the average taxpayer may consider to be 'splitting hairs'. Thus, a GP who buys suits to use in his consulting room would be unable to obtain any tax relief for that expenditure because the Revenue considers suits to be primarily for a private purpose with some incidental element of practice use. On the other hand, the same principle is unlikely to be applied to such expenses as motoring costs, the Inland Revenue fully accepting the element of practice use as allowable.

The attitude of the Inland Revenue

Historically, GPs have received relatively generous treatment from the Inland Revenue in the scrutiny of their expenses claims. However, there has been a change of approach in recent years. There is some evidence that the accounts and claims of self-employed GPs, both medical and dental, have been subject to particularly close examination and that Inspectors of Taxes have queried such claims under a number of headings.

Experience has shown that claims for salaries paid to spouses, motor expenses, practice use of houses and telephone costs are particularly vulnerable. The inclusion of estimates is also penalized in some cases. It is in the power of the Inland Revenue to investigate past tax years, and this new, more stringent, attitude has been very costly for a few unfortunate GPs.

Where the Inland Revenue is able to establish a pattern of over-claiming lasting for several years, it is empowered to increase assessments retrospectively, possibly over as much as six years, seeking to collect not only lost tax, but also interest and penalties. It is essential that GPs making claims for expenses, and discussing with their accountants the manner in which these are formulated, should understand the risk of unrealistic claims instigating an in-depth investigation. In particular, it should be ensured that:

1 all claims submitted are clearly justified and that the expenditure has been made for practice purposes
2 receipts are available to support all claims
3 where restrictions for private use are in force, they can be justified
4 claims showing estimated expenditure are avoided so far as is possible. Where these are unavoidable, the fact that they are estimates should be clearly shown on the claims submitted to the Inland Revenue.

GPs should understand that, when a claim is prepared on their behalf by an accountant, the onus is upon them to keep the accountant informed of genuine expenses incurred *and* to check draft claims before submission in order to ensure that no unjustified or incorrect claims are made. The GP should be asked to sign the claim as correct before it is submitted to the Inland Revenue.

What can be claimed?

Claims can fall under a number of general headings.

1 Expenditure paid personally by the GP but which can clearly be demonstrated as being solely for practice purposes, such as medical equipment, medical journals and subscriptions.
2 Expenses incurred for partially practice and partially private use, such as home telephone and motoring.

3 Expenses for which the GP wishes to claim but can produce no receipts or invoices, and estimates, may be submitted. However, as has been outlined above, claims of this nature are particularly at risk of attracting unwanted Revenue attention.

GPs frequently ask 'What claims am I entitled to make?'. In short, they have no entitlement to claim anything; indeed claiming an expense and having it allowed by the Revenue are two separate matters. A GP can look for ever at the Income Tax Acts and will find no reference to doctors' cars, houses and the like. Over-claiming on expenditure and hoping that the Inland Revenue will allow it is unprofessional, and the penalties for over-claiming can be serious.

The preparation of such claims can cause dissent between the GP and the accountant. An accountant who advises his client to moderate claims to a level which will be acceptable to the Inland Revenue, yet which do not deprive the GP of any tax relief to which he might legitimately be due, is attempting to protect his client in advance from an Inland Revenue enquiry. The accountant is acting in the long-term interests of the GP, and the latter should accept advice of this nature.

Who should submit the claim?

In the rare case of a GP who does not engage an accountant, that GP will submit and formulate a claim, agreeing this with the Inland Revenue. This approach may not be in the best interests of the GP, who has no specialist knowledge in dealing with local Inspectors of Taxes. Tax returns are better left to a professional accountant who is an expert at negotiations of this nature.

If the GP is in a single-handed practice, the claim would normally be produced as part of the practice accounts without the necessity for submitting separate claims, and no undue difficulty would arise in this case. However, in the case of GPs in partnerships, problems can arise concerning who is to prepare the claim.

In some partnerships, the GPs choose to have separate accountants to deal with their personal affairs. This is their prerogative (see Chapter 49), but it should be accepted that the accountant who deals with the partnership may have a superior knowledge of the negotiations which have been conducted with the Inspector of Taxes and there are excellent reasons for the same accountant to act for all the partners in submitting personal expenses claims. The accountant may be able to obtain some sort of omnibus agreement from the Inland Revenue to the partners' advantage and only if he is acting for all the partners in a practice can they take full advantage of this.

The submission of claims by separate accountants may well be done on different bases and, even if only one of these claims provokes an enquiry from the Inland Revenue, this may spread to encompass all the GPs in the partnership.

Practice use of home

The majority of GPs use their home to a greater or lesser degree for practice purposes. Some GPs have no central surgery, and some single-handed practitioners have a surgery in part of their house. Such doctors have a legitimate claim for a major share of the costs of running the house. At the other end of the scale, GPs living several miles away from the practice area, who use their homes mainly for occasional study or reference purposes, cannot make claims on the same basis.

Proportion of running expenses

Claims are frequently made for practice use of GPs' houses, based upon the proportion which the practice use of the house bears to the total floor area, or by some similar means. Such claims, possibly when extended to include qualifying repairs expenditure and excess mortgage interest, can be substantial.

To ensure that such claims are justified, they should be made only when:

1 there is clear evidence of the use of the house for consulting or treatment of patients on a regular basis
2 a professional plate is displayed outside the house (although not mandatory, this could make the acceptance of a borderline claim more likely)
3 there is an appropriate entry in the local telephone directory
4 the house is either within, or adjacent to, the practice area.

If the claim is to be fully justified, point 1 must apply.

Having established that the basis for such a claim exists, it is necessary to calculate the fractional cost of the total house expenses to be claimed. The method usually employed, and which is invariably acceptable to the Inland Revenue, is to award an arbitrary points figure to every room in the house, more or less dependent upon its size, and then to allocate those points between practice and private use (*see* Figure 41.1). For instance, if there is a study where patients are seen and which is used for no other purpose, all of the points attributable to this room can be allocated to practice use. Conversely, it is unlikely that an upstairs bedroom or bathroom can be allocated other than wholly for private use. This system may be based on floor areas, but this may be felt to be an over-complication.

The expenses included in the claim should be the normal running costs of the house, *excluding* capital expenditure.

Figure 41.2 shows a worked example of a typical claim for a GP's house expenses, with none of the rooms used exclusively for practice use, but which finally gives a fractional figure of one-seventh to be claimed. Although the principle of this method is likely to be acceptable to an Inspector of Taxes, the allocation of the various rooms may be negotiable.

Study allowance

Where the house is not regularly used for consultations, but the GP spends time working at home, it is much less contentious to claim a 'study allowance',

Dr B Truman, 'Watneys', 19 Courage Road, Worthington-on-Bass

	Practice	Private	Total
Downstairs:			
Garage (double)	12	8	20
Kitchen	1	14	15
Lounge (waiting)	2	18	20
Dining room	–	15	15
Study (consulting)	7	3	10
Entrance hall	1	4	5
Cloakroom	1	4	5
Storage room	1	4	5
Upstairs:			
Main bedroom	–	20	20
3 bedrooms (15 each)	–	45	45
Bathroom	–	10	10
WC	–	5	5
	25	150	175

Figure 41.1 Practice proportion of private house expenses: 'points' system

Practice proportion of private house expenses

House expenses	£
Rent	–
Council tax	825
Lighting and heating	892
Repairs and renewals*	598
Window cleaning	65
Insurance	150
Domestic assistance (£10 per week)	520
Garden expenses (1/4 of £1 000—subject to negotiation)	250
	3300
Claim: one-seventh	471

* includes: £200 interior decorating; £150 electrical repairs;
£225 part (half) cost of replacement windows.

Figure 41.2   A house expenses claim

based on a lump sum estimate of the additional cost to the GP of using the house for that purpose. A typical annual claim might be £1 per hour for 10 hours per week over 46 weeks a year, ie £460. Alternatively, a round sum per week could be claimed.

Community charge, business rate and council tax

Those GPs who previously claimed a domestic rates bill will not have been able to claim the community charge, or 'poll tax'. However, they may find themselves liable to a proportion of the new business rate if part of their house is used exclusively for practice purposes. In some cases, GPs may be able to claim a refund of these rates from the NHS. They will also be able to claim the new council tax which, like the domestic rates, is a tax based on property.

Capital gains tax

One factor that frequently deters GPs from making a claim for house expenses is that they have been advised that, in the event of the house being sold at a profit at some time in the future, they will be liable for capital gains tax on a proportion of the gain realized.

This is *not* the case; in such circumstances, capital gains tax will not be charged unless part of the house was used exclusively for practice purposes. Even if this were the case, if the doctor acquired a replacement house also used in his practice, it is likely that 'roll-over' relief could be claimed.

It is highly unlikely that a GP selling a house which has been partially used in his practice will give rise to an actual charge upon which capital gains tax is payable.

The subject of capital gains tax on GPs' houses is extremely complex and specialist professional advice should always be sought. No GP should be dissuaded from making a legitimate claim for house expenses merely by the prospect of having to pay capital gains tax at some time in the future.

Other practice expenses

Apart from private use of houses, other main items included in the claim are discussed in other chapters: motor expenses in Chapter 42 and spouses' salaries in Chapter 43. However, there are many other expenses that can and should be claimed by GPs where justified.

There is some evidence of substantial under-claiming by GPs for other expenses. It is important that they are claimed fully, not only for the purpose of reducing the GP's tax liability, but also to ensure that a full record of expenses is available in practice accounts submitted to the Inland Revenue and which may be included in the sampling process from which the GP's pay award is calculated.

Other such claims may include the following.

- *Medical subscriptions.* All GPs pay their registration fee to the GMC and will subscribe also to one of the medical defence organizations. They may also be members of the BMA, RCGP and several other societies of a more specific nature within the profession. Care should be taken to see that all these subscriptions and levies are properly recorded and claimed.
- *Charitable and other donations.* Some GPs make donations of a medico-charitable nature and, provided these are of a reasonable amount, the local Inspector of Taxes will allow them against profits. Again these should be properly recorded.
- *Medical books and journals.* Although GPs receive much literature free of charge, some subscribe regularly to medical journals, as well as purchasing books for reference purposes. All payments of this nature should be properly recorded and claimed.

- *Locum fees, etc.* Many GPs make payments to locums for temporarily looking after their practice, as well as payments for deputizing and relief services. In many cases, depending largely on clauses in the partnership deed, these may be made personally by the partners rather than out of partnership funds.
- *Security expenses.* As many GPs keep valuable drugs and equipment in their houses, the necessity for expenditure on some form of security is obvious. A proportion of the cost of installing burglar alarms, their annual maintenance and the provision of security locks should be claimed for tax purposes.
- *Bank charges.* GPs often use their private bank account to some degree for practice purposes, for example, by paying part of their house costs, motor expenses and other sundry items from their private account. If a charge is made by the bank for use of this account, a proportion of the charges (but not interest) can be included in the claim.
- *Cleaning and laundry.* Most of this expense is likely to be paid from the partnership, but if privately paid, the laundry of overalls, protective clothing and the like should be claimed. Claims for the cleaning of normal wear, such as suits and dresses, is unlikely to be accepted unless a particularly good case can be made. Claims for the purchase of such ordinary items of clothing will not be allowed under any circumstances.
- *Medical instruments.* The upkeep of medical equipment is a proper claim and all amounts, eg for cleaning or replacements, should be carefully listed and included under this heading.
- *Waiting room papers and flowers.* This is often included in overall house expenses and reduced accordingly. It is preferable to claim this as a separate entity if justified.
- *Accountancy fees.* Most of the practice accountancy bills will be paid from partnership funds but, if any charges are made to individual GPs for personal expenses claims, etc, these should be claimed. No claim can be made, however the bill is paid, for dealing with a GP's personal income tax return.
- *Insurance premiums.* The insurance on the house will normally be included in a house expenses claim. Motor insurance should be included in the claim for car expenses. However, a few premiums can be included under general practice expenses; namely public liability insurance and insurance of medical and surgical equipment.

  Life assurance payments do not qualify for relief, nor do payments of sickness and permanent health insurance premiums, including 'locum insurance'. However, if there is a claim on the health policy, the benefit will not be taxed as a receipt unless this continues for more than one year.

- *Courses and conferences.* In many cases, costs of attending courses are refunded from NHS sources and, where no net cost is met by the GP, obviously no claim can be made.

  However, other conferences attended at the GP's own expense can be claimed for, although difficulty may be experienced in having claims for major overseas conferences accepted. If the GP is accompanied by a spouse, the Inspector of Taxes is likely to insist that his or her share of the costs is excluded from the claim.
- *Private telephone bills.* In some partnerships, it is the policy of the practice that all private telephone accounts are paid from partnership funds. However, in other cases, these will be met personally and an agreed proportion of the cost of the calls should be included in the claim. This will be a matter of record and negotiation. Some Inspectors of Taxes will also allow a proportion of the rental charge. VAT is included on private telephone bills and this should be claimed too.
- *Photographic expenses.* Many GPs use cameras for medical reasons, often in connection with training purposes. This is a reasonable claim to make, although some element of private use may have to be taken into account.
- *Maintenance of approach.* The cost of maintaining the garden and surroundings of a house used for practice purposes can be claimed in several ways. Part of the cost of the upkeep of the approach to the house, to the extent that it is likely to be used by patients, is a proper claim, either by inclusion in an overall claim for house expenses, or separately.
- *Computers and technical equipment.* The use by GPs of personally owned computers, video equipment, etc, is increasing. Where such equipment is bought and retained in the GP's private house, some difficulty may be experienced in having the claim agreed, as they are likely to be used to a large degree for private and recreational purposes. If, however, such equipment were to be bought by the practice and included as a partnership asset retained in the surgery, little difficulty is likely to be encountered.

Summary

It is assumed that GPs will spend on average £22 190 on their practice expenses in the year ending 31 March 1994. This figure, which is worked out annually by the Doctors' and Dentists' Review Body, is based on GP accounts and claims submitted to the Inland Revenue, and may undervalue the total amount spent.

If a GP spends less than this, both through his partnership and by way of personal expenses claims, he may not be claiming all that he should.

42 Cars and Motoring

VIRTUALLY all GPs use their car to a greater or lesser degree for practice purposes. There is little difficulty in obtaining tax relief on part of the expenses thus incurred. However, the manner in which the proportion to be claimed is to be calculated is a matter of negotiation between the accountant, his GP client and the Inspector of Taxes.

Type of car

There is no restriction on the type of vehicle upon which allowances can be claimed. Claims can and have been allowed on Land Rovers, motor and pedal cycles. In theory, it is not of undue concern whether the doctor runs a Rolls Royce or a Mini (but beware of the expensive cars rule, *see* page 253); the expenses will be allowed and calculated on the same basis.

What expenses can be claimed?

The claim should include all amounts spent during the year of account in running, maintaining and servicing the car. Estimates should be avoided. Such expenses are likely to cover:

- road fund licence
- motor insurance premiums
- MOT tests
- petrol and oil
- repairs and servicing
- interest on loan finance (which may be restricted)
- hire purchase interest
- car parking
- car washing charges
- AA/RAC subscriptions.

It is essential that all receipts are retained for inspection if required.

Other travelling expenses

Other forms of travel can be claimed where relevant, usually without any restriction for private use, where amounts have been specifically spent on business use. These may include such items as taxi, train and bus fares.

Calculating the 'private use' element

The most contentious part of preparing and agreeing claims of this nature is determining the element of private use which has to be taken into account before the Inland Revenue will accept the claim as allowable for income tax purposes.

Rarely are GPs' cars genuinely used 100% for practice purposes. For the most part, the car which is the subject of a claim will be used both for practice and private purposes. The Inland Revenue rule is that travel between home and surgery is considered as private use; the car that the GP uses for his rounds will almost certainly travel from home to the surgery and back at least once a day and this cannot be treated as practice use.

The Inland Revenue tend to be hard on claims which are not prepared logically, ie by assuming a claim of 95% without any evidence to support this. Claims formulated in this way are often the subject of enquiries by the Inland Revenue and possibly of claims for arrears of tax, interest and penalties.

To establish business mileage, it is often advisable to keep detailed records of mileage for a specimen period of not less than two months, allocated between practice and private use. This can be summarized and the two factors added together to produce an agreed proportion. A typical example of the calculation of a mileage log kept for a period of two months is set out in Figure 42.1.

More than one car

GPs frequently ask whether they will be able to claim tax relief on more than one car. There is no reason why not, as long as reasonable claims are submitted, which can be substantiated in the normal manner. Major claims should be made for the principal practice car and minor claims for the second car, such as:

First car   80%
Second car   30%

If claiming for two cars , it is desirable to maintain a regular mileage log (*see* Figure 42.1).

It is not sufficient merely to have a second car available for use as required or in emergencies; a claim can only be entirely valid if the GP can demonstrate at least some regular practice use.

Expensive cars

The Inland Revenue define an expensive car as one costing over £12 000. This limit was increased from £8000, in respect of cars purchased from 10 March 1992.

Dr John Wilson and his wife Mary each run a car, both of which are used to some degree in his medical practice. John has been advised by his accountants to keep a detailed mileage log for each car for a specimen period of two months in order that his proportion of private use can be accurately calculated. Both John and Mary produce weekly mileage figures which, when collated, show the following results.

Mileage logs: June/July 1993

| | John [Rover] Miles | | | Mary [Mini] Miles | | |
	Total	*Practice*	*Private*	*Total*	*Practice*	*Private*
Week ended:						
June 5	475	420	55	63	20	43
12	125	50	75	385	195	190
19	578	300	278	75	15	60
26	487	400	87	88	8	80
July 3	569	525	44	56	16	40
10	87	20	67	468	170	298
17	625	557	68	42	24	18
24	480	404	76	50	38	12
31	360	350	10	68	34	34
Total (2 months)	3786	3026	760	1295	520	775
Percentages		79.9	20.1		40.2	59.8

From this log it would seem that John could justify a practice claim for 80% of the Rover (20% restriction) and for 40% of the Mini (60% restriction).

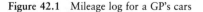

Figure 42.1 Mileage log for a GP's cars

If a car is bought for an amount in excess of this figure, the capital allowances (*see* below) are calculated as if the car had cost £12 000.

This restriction also applies to claims for interest relief on the cost of financing the purchase. This will normally be scaled down proportionately. If a GP leases a car, any tax relief he might claim for leasing charges will be similarly reduced.

Tax allowances for depreciation

GPs will be granted an annual capital allowance ('writing-down allowance') on the cost or written-down value of the car, amounting to 25% per annum.

If a car is sold, a GP will receive a balancing allowance if the sale price is less than the written down value, or be subject to a balancing charge if it is greater.

Examples of two separate car purchases, one of these an expensive car costing over £12 000, are shown in Figure 42.2. At the end of the lives of the

	Dr John Leech	
	Bloggs Banger *D436TGM*	*Super Road-Hog* *J639ABC*
Accounting year-end: 30 June		
Banger, bought April 1992	7000	
Road-Hog, bought June 1992		15 500
Writing-down allowance 1993/94 (25%)	1750	3000 *
	5250	12 500
Writing-down allowance, 1994/95 (25%)+	1312	3000 *
	3938	9500
Writing-down allowance, 1995/96 (25%)+	984	2375
	2954	7125
Banger sold: December 1994	2750	
Road-Hog sold: March 1995		8250
Balancing allowance: 1996/97+	204	
Balancing charge: 1996/97+		(1125)

*Restricted allowance
+Tax calculations for 1995/96 and onwards may be affected by change to actual year basis of assessment.
In practice, all claims will be reduced by agreed proportion of private use.

Figure 42.2   Capital allowances on cars

cars they are sold by the GP, one of them giving rise to a balancing allowance and one to a balancing charge. In the case of the expensive car, the annual writing-down allowance is limited to what it would have been had the original cost of the car been £12 000.

All claims, including the annual allowance, balancing allowance and balancing charge, will in practice be reduced by the amount of the agreed element of private use. Thus, if in our example Dr Leech has agreed he will claim 80% expenses on his 'Super Road-Hog', the allowance for the 1994/95 year of £3000 would be reduced to £2400.

The granting of capital allowances on these cars works the same way as expenses are claimed and profits assessed for tax purposes, ie on a preceding year basis. Therefore, from the illustration, Dr Leech makes up his accounts to 30 June 1992 so that these would first be allowed for tax purposes in the 1994/95 tax year.

Timing of purchase

Many GPs ask what is the best time for them to change their car for tax reasons. However, there are many reasons for changing cars, not all of them financial. A car may be several years old and expensive in terms of repairs and parts; in these circumstances, it may be sensible to dispose of the car for whatever it will fetch, regardless of timing.

In general, though, a GP would be well advised to change a car immediately before his financial year-end. Again, taking the illustration, if Dr Leech wishes to change his car he should do so in June rather than July each year. This will mean, by application of the preceding year principle, that he will receive the first annual allowance for that car a year earlier. Thus, if he bought the car in June 1992 as he did, he would get the allowance in the 1993/94 tax year. Had he delayed the purchase for a few weeks and bought it in early July, he would not have received the first tax allowance until the 1994/95 year.

Financing the purchase

Few GPs can afford to buy their cars without recourse to some means of finance. There is a clear scale of preferred means of acquiring a car, the order of which is shown below.

1 Outright purchase without recourse to borrowing.

2 Free (or low) loan from motor dealer or agent (usually requiring substantial deposit).
3 Bank (business development) loan.
4 Hire purchase.
5 Leasing.

The first institution approached by a GP wishing to borrow money to finance a new car should be his bank. Hopefully, he will be regarded as a good credit risk and the bank should be able to offer a fixed interest loan, probably a business development loan, upon which the interest will remain constant for the two- or three-year period. Loans of this nature should not extend to a date later than the anticipated life of the car.

Buying or leasing

There has been much comment in recent years over GPs leasing cars for use in their practice and obtaining tax relief on the premiums. Experience shows that the overall cost of leasing is likely to be greater than the monthly cost of buying a car under a bank loan or hire purchase.

It is difficult to generalize because there are numerous types of leasing contracts, many of which involve variations in payments for repairs and running costs and, above all, the conditions on which the car might be transferred to the lessee after the contract period. Each scheme must therefore be evaluated separately and considered on its merits.

GPs, by virtue of their exempt status for VAT (*see* Chapter 45), are unable to recover the VAT charged by the leasing company on the monthly charges. This greatly increases the cost to the GP and, for that reason, the leasing of cars by GPs is not generally considered to be financially viable. Some practices may, however, be able to register for VAT under the partial exemption rules (*see* page 268).

Tax saving on cars

There is likely to be a private use restriction on any tax relief claimed on cars, according to the cirumstances of the GP concerned. However, provided the normal rules are adhered to, the treatment of GPs' cars for tax purposes is not ungenerous. It is worth emphasizing that necessary and normal expenditure on cars can be an excellent and useful method of tax saving, as long as all expenditure is recorded, all bills are retained and a full and accurate claim is prepared. A methodical system of recording such expenditure is vital.

Finally, it is *not* financially efficient to buy and sell cars purely for the tax relief. The cost of buying a new car is far more than a GP would receive in tax relief, which should be regarded as an incidental benefit.

43 Spouses and Families

THIS chapter considers the financial aspects of the part which the GP's spouse and family play in his or her practice.

Despite the age of sex equality, and more recently the introduction of separate tax assessments for husbands and wives, the majority of GPs are still men, who may be married with several children. This chapter initially concentrates on them, and then, later in the chapter, the case of married women GPs is considered.

A wife's salary

The facility for male GPs to pay a salary to their wives is an excellent if limited means of tax saving. In effect, a salary can be paid up to a prescribed level to the wife for certain qualifying duties. This salary will qualify as a tax-allowable expense, by its inclusion in the GP's own claim for personal practice expenses and, provided she has no other income, the salary will be free of tax in the hands of the recipient.

It is standard practice to maintain this salary at a level below the threshold at which Class 1 National Insurance contributions (*see* Chapter 44) come into force, to avoid the payment of these contributions both by the wife, as the employee, and the husband as the employer. The payment of such contributions would diminish any tax relief available to the husband.

For the 1994/95 tax year the threshold at which Class 1 National Insurance comes into force is £57 weekly, which works out at £2964 per annum or £242 per calendar month. It is therefore suggested that the level of the wife's salary be kept at a level no higher than £245 monthly.

For 1995/96 the threshold will rise to £59 per week and the salary should be maintained at a level no higher than £254 per month.

Qualifying duties

In order to ensure that the payment of the wife's salary will not be questioned by the Inland Revenue, she should be performing duties commensurate with the payment made. The duties typically include:

- telephone answering
- secretarial and reception duties

- chauffeuring
- book-keeping, including signature of cheques
- chaperoning.

In some cases, it may be possible for other duties to be performed, depending on the wife's professional qualifications.

Should a payment be made?

To ensure that the salary is acceptable to the Inland Revenue, a payment should be made by the physical transfer of funds, ideally as a monthly cheque drawn on the husband's bank account in favour of the wife. Some couples, however, have joint bank accounts and in these cases it may be preferable for either a cash cheque in favour of the wife to be drawn or for a separate account to be opened in the wife's name and the salary paid into that account. However the salary is paid, there *must* be evidence of a physical transfer of funds.

Payment by partnerships

Partnerships frequently seek to pay out salaries of this nature to the wives of male GPs from partnership funds. This is not recommended, because it is rare for a partnership to be made up of married male GPs only. Other GPs in the practice may be single or married women to whom a salary payment is not suitable. It could therefore be unfair if these salaries are paid from partnership funds and taken into account before the partnership profits are allocated. In addition, some of the partners may have chosen to pension their wives (*see* below); it is unlikely that they will all be of the same age and attract identical pension contributions. Again, unfairness can result if pensions are paid from partnership funds.

For these reasons, it is suggested that wives' salaries should be paid by the husbands for whom they will largely be working, except in the case of wives who work in the surgery on a regular basis.

A wife who has outside employment

Frequently, wives of younger GPs tend to have outside employment, and it is often assumed that in these cases a wife's salary should not be paid. This is not the case. If a wife earns sufficient income from her outside job to cover her personal allowance, there will be no tax benefit to the family unit concerned.

Neither can there be any loss, unless the wife is paying a higher rate of tax than her husband. In such a case, a salary cannot be beneficial and should not be paid. In most cases, however, a salary can be paid, if only to maintain a precedent. A wife may choose to leave her outside employment and the salary would then become of great benefit.

Wives' pension plans

A further means of tax saving is to take out a pension scheme for a wife employed in her husband's practice. The premiums paid under such a policy are allowable deductions for income tax purposes and the husband will receive tax relief for them. Upon retirement the pension arising from such a policy will be treated as earned income for the wife. Such pension policies should be the priority means of investment from income by the GP concerned.

The Inland Revenue has in a few cases judged the level of salary paid to the wife upon the basis of the total payment, that is to say the salary and pension premiums combined. It is therefore even more important to ensure that the salary upon which the pension is based, is paid for service provided, at a realistic rate of remuneration paid on a regular basis.

Married women doctors

A married woman GP can pay a salary to her husband, provided the payment can be justified by using the criteria above. However, there is little point in the wife who is taxed at 25% (if part-time) paying a salary to her husband if he pays tax at 40% on the same money. Where the husband has no income, is a pensioner or paying tax at a low rate, a spouse's salary may be appropriate.

Payments to children

A GP's family unit may include responsible teenagers who can do some of the work which the wife of a married male GP often performs, such as reception/telephone answering duties. If this is the case, a realistic salary can be paid to the children concerned.

Medical insurance premiums

Where premiums are paid by the doctor for a policy of medical insurance to his spouse (BUPA, PPP, etc) these can also be included in an expenses claim. Only the premium that relates to the spouse should be paid. In some circumstances, GPs may take out a separate policy in the spouse's name or, in the case of a family policy, the overall premium may be apportioned.

44 National Insurance Contributions

NATIONAL Insurance is sometimes called 'the hidden income tax' because it receives relatively little publicity and changes made are not normally announced in each year's Budget. This system is likely to change, however, following the introduction of November budgets from 1993.

National Insurance contributions (NIC) can account for a surprisingly large slice of a GP's income. There are four main classes of insurance which may apply to a greater or lesser degree to most GPs.

Class 1 contributions

Class 1 NIC contributions are paid by deduction from an employee's wage or salary. The rates are calculated by means of contribution tables and paid over to the Inland Revenue by the employer each month, together with the staff PAYE deductions.

Some employees, notably GP trainees, are 'contracted out' of the NHS scheme, which means that they are part of an employers' scheme and consequently pay lower contributions.

GPs, as employers, are in many cases able to recover 100% of their share of NICs for ancillary staff from the FHSA.

Class 2 contributions

Class 2 contributions are paid by self-employed people, including GPs. Since April 1993 these contributions are paid by a system of quarterly billings by the Contribution Agency who are responsible for the collection of NICs. There is also a facility for payment by direct debit, either from the personal account of the doctor concerned or from a partnership account. The system of paying these contributions by stamping a card was abolished from 12 April 1993. Such contributions are the personal liability of the doctor concerned and are not an item of partnership expenses; they should be charged to his current account.

GPs who pay Class 2 NIC by either of the above methods should ensure that they obtain credit for weeks when contributions are not payable, either through sickness or a period of unemployment.

Class 3 contributions

Class 3 contributions are paid by non-employed people, usually to protect their rights to a state retirement pension. These are frequently paid by men who retire before the age of 65 years and who have not made a sufficient contribution during their working lives to qualify for a full pension. Payment is on the same basis as for Class 2.

Class 4 contributions

Class 4 contributions are paid on a band of income which changes from year to year. In the 1993/94 year, earnings falling within this band of income are assessed at 6.3% and the maximum amount which can be paid by any contributor is £976.50.

Registration

The practice manager is strongly advised to ensure that all GPs in the practice have a National Insurance record. New partners should approach their local DSS office to register for this purpose; otherwise arrears of contributions may be charged. Alternatively, GPs can register for NICs by writing to:

The Contribution Agency
Class 2 Group
Department of Social Security
Longbenton
Newcastle-upon-Tyne NE98 14X

In addition, there is a freephone enquiry line (0800 393539).
Rates of contributions for the 1993/94 year are set out in Appendix C.

Deferment

Some GPs will be required to contribute to three separate classes of National Insurance: 1, 2 and 4. Classes 2 and 4 are required because they are self-employed taxpayers and Class 1 will be paid by GPs who take appointments at local hospitals. In these cases, it is possible to obtain a deferment of

Class 4 and in some cases Class 2 contributions where it is evident that the GP will pay in excess of the annual maximum.

Deferment is applied for by submission of form CF359 to the National Insurance office by 5 April in each tax year. Where deferment is obtained, but the eventual contributions under Classes 1, 2 and 4 are insufficient to meet an annual maximum figure, a demand for unpaid contributions will be issued, probably for several years in arrears.

Repayment

Where, on the other hand, contributions for a single year are overpaid, a repayment will be sent to the contributor. In the case of a partnership, it is important, to ensure fairness, that the payment is credited to the partner who paid the original contribution.

45 Value Added Tax

As of December 1994, radical changes in the way in which VAT is assessed under the schemes outlined below are pending and this chapter should be read with this in mind. (*See also* note on page x.)

VAT was introduced in the early 1970s, as part of the Treaty of Rome through which the UK became a member of the European Community. However, the supply of services by a registered medical practitioner (which for this purpose includes dentists and allied services) is exempt from VAT as one of several exemptions involving health care professions in general.

In practice, this means that a GP, regardless of his level of earnings, is not required to register for VAT. Although a GP is not required to add VAT to fees to patients, he cannot recover the input tax on such items upon which VAT is chargeable, which include:

- professional fees
- telephone charges
- petrol and car servicing
- supply of certain medical equipment
- equipment leasing charges
- fees for courses and conferences
- stationery bills
- gas and electricity bills.

For the majority of expenses in a typical GP's accounts, no VAT is chargeable, eg staff salaries, rent and rates, loan interest and charges, insurance premiums, life insurance and pension contributions.

It would appear that a GP suffers by the operation of this rule, ie by incurring an extra 17.5% charged on a proportion of his practice expenses that cannot be recovered from any source. However, it should also be borne in mind that these total expenses are included in the practice accounts as items of expenditure, upon which the annual Review Body award is based (*see* Chapter 3), and as such they are, albeit indirectly, refunded.

If GPs run other businesses, this exemption does not extend to any trading carried on outside their medical practice or where VAT-chargeable supplies are involved.

Figure 45.1 shows the changes that have occurred in VAT rules as they affect GPs over the last 20 years.

1974	VAT introduced in the UK. Supply of medical services exempt.
1984	VAT extended to building alterations and extensions. No increase in cost rent limits.
1988	Decision in European Court: VAT to be levied on new building constructions.
April 1989	VAT levied on contractors' bills for new developments. Separate cost rent limits introduced.
August 1989	Self-supply rule introduced. GPs required to register in certain cases.
January 1992	Self-supply principle extended to surgery extensions.
April 1992	Partial exemption rule extended to GPs and certain other professions.
June 1993	VAT added by FHSAs to determine cost rent reimbursements.

Figure 45.1   VAT and the GP: timetable of events

Surgery developments and the 'self-supply' rule

The history of surgery developments and their involvement with VAT began in the mid-1980s. When VAT was introduced in 1974, no charge was levied on any building work of the type usually undertaken by GPs and no undue problems arose. In 1984, however, the Government extended the scope of VAT to include alterations and extensions to existing buildings. This applies to GPs who embark upon schemes of enlargement of their surgeries or who buy a property for re-development into a new surgery. Cost rent limits were not extended to include the VAT charge, so GPs who develop and renovate existing buildings are unable to claim a cost rent limit which reflects the true amount paid.

In 1988 the European Court ruled that in future VAT would have to be levied on new building constructions. This causes problems for trades and professions, including GPs, who are unable to register for VAT. This ruling came into effect on 1 April 1989, and from that date, the cost rent limits were increased to reflect the higher VAT charge on the construction costs. No similar arrangement was made in respect of building alterations, and rates A and B still apply to these building cost limits.

A self-supply charge was introduced on 1 August 1989 by which doctors are treated as 'developers' for VAT purposes if they:

- construct a building
- order a building to be constructed
- finance the construction of a building with a view to selling, leasing, occupying or using all or part of it.

As developers, they become liable to a self-supply charge if they lease out any part of the building on a VAT exempt basis, or use it in connection with an exempt business activity, including medical practice, within 10 years of completion.

The self-supply rule applies to constructions commenced on or after 1 August 1989, where the building and land costs, including professional fees and fittings but excluding bridging interest (*see* page 171), exceed £100 000. Wherever this charge applies, the practice is required to register and account for VAT on the completion date. However, the practice may register as an 'intending trader' as soon as there is evidence that the development will go ahead, which is normally after planning permission has been granted. The advantage of registering early is that the VAT incurred may be recovered during the construction period, providing a cash flow benefit. VAT incurred on any services related to the construction in the six-month period prior to registering may also be recovered. However, if any VAT is recovered on a scheme which subsequently proves to be abortive, a refund must be made.

Other expenses on which VAT is incurred are subject to the VAT partial exemption rules (*see* below). The VAT must be accounted for on goods and services subject to VAT in their own right, such as travel packs and earnings from writing and lecturing, after registration on quarterly VAT returns which must be submitted within 30 days of a period-end to avoid any penalties.

Applications for VAT registration should be made on form VAT 1, which is available from all local VAT offices. The application should be accompanied by a letter explaining the reason for registration, ie to account for the self-supply charge. Intending trader registrants must also enclose evidence that the development will take place, eg a copy of the planning permission.

The VAT self-supply charge is 17.5% of the total cost of construction and acquiring the land, together with professional fees incurred. As VAT is always payable on construction costs and architect's fees etc, the real additional cost is the VAT charge arising from the cost of acquiring the land. Thus, the practice is required to pay VAT on the purchase price of the development land and the VAT self-supply charge.

Surgery extensions and reconstructions

The VAT self-supply charge was extended from 1 January 1992 to include some extensions of existing surgeries. In these cases, the project must be registered for VAT if the extended building uses land outside the bounds of the previous building. If the GPs have owned at least 75% of all the land (newly and existing) for 10 years prior to the extension being completed, the self-supply charge will not arise. In cases where the extension or enlargement increases the building floor area by 20% or more, the self-supply charge is based on the cost of the works and land proportionate to the increase in floor area.

The self-supply charge on surgery reconstructions applies to work commenced after 1 January 1992, where the total cost is more than £100 000, and which involve the removal of 80% or more of the floor structure.

VAT and cost rent reimbursements

When the self-supply rule was imposed in 1989, it was unclear whether the full VAT cost should be included in the total cost upon which cost rent reimbursement was calculated (*see* Figure 28.2, page 171). This was to a large degree resolved by the introduction of revised arrangements from June 1993, whereby FHSAs will add VAT, where incurred, to total costs. GPs now developing new surgeries should add the VAT to their total cost and it will then be included in their cost rent reimbursement. This does not, however, extend to building alterations and extensions, to which the lower rate B (*see* Appendix F) will continue to apply.

Partial exemption and the 'de minimis' rule

New VAT regulations introduced from 1 April 1992 give businesses partial exemption from VAT. General practices can reclaim the VAT on their costs and overheads, subject to their being able to display an element of VATable income and that the VAT on their costs and overheads does not exceed £7200 per annum (£600 per month). When this rule was introduced, a number of practices were successful in registering with their local VAT offices, but in October 1992 Customs and Excise suspended new VAT registrations for NHS doctors and dentists. This was contested by the Department of Health and in March 1993 Customs and Excise were compelled to reverse their ruling.

A practice seeking to recover VAT must take care that the total VAT paid out in a single year does not exceed £7200, which represents, at a VAT rate of 17.5%, a total chargeable expenditure of £41 142; otherwise no repayment will be forthcoming.

It is necessary, when registering for VAT, to display an element of income which is derived from sources outside medical work and which is normally subject to VAT. Where registration is accepted, a practice must be prepared to make quarterly VAT returns and to pay VAT on the income earned from these sources. Where possible, eg in the case of such items as passport applications and private prescriptions, a GP must be prepared to add VAT at the rate currently in force when a charge is made. The major items which fall into this category are shown in Figure 45.2.

- Royalties.
- Lecturing fees.
- Articles for publication.
- Retainer fees (non-medical).
- Passport authentication fees.
- Private prescriptions.
- Proceeds from pay phones, coffee machines, etc.
- Fees for travel packs, condoms, etc.
- Advertising fees, eg from advertisements on posters in the waiting room and in-practrice leaflets.
- PGEA meeting charges.

Figure 45.2   Examples of VATable income in general practice

Experience has shown that medium sized practices are likely to benefit most from these rules. The small partnership or single-handed practice may be unable to justify a large enough repayment to cover the work entailed, whilst the larger practice, say of eight or more doctors, is likely to have total expenses above the limit of £7200.

VAT on drugs

GPs who dispense drugs, either from full dispensing practices or by the supply of occasional items such as influenza vaccines, pay VAT to the drug supplier. Those practices are not required to register for VAT, which is recovered in effect through the standard drugs tariff. (*See also* Chapter 33.)

However, where a practice employs a registered pharmacist, the dispensing of drugs is subject to VAT at the zero rate. The practice can therefore register and reclaim the VAT on the purchase of the drugs from Customs and Excise. The PPA will then reimburse the practice for the cost of the drugs, exclusive of VAT.

Where a non-dispensing practice registers for VAT under these rules, the drugs administered by the GP are part of his exempt services. He can reclaim the VAT on the drugs, together with all other VAT on costs and overheads, as indicated above. The inclusion of such VAT on items of practice expense could, however, push the practice over the 'de minimis' limit.

46 Insurance

ONE of several professional advisers the GP may consult during his working life is the insurance broker. However, many doctors do not use a single broker but buy policies on a random basis, often without any overall planning.

Constant, regular and knowledgeable insurance advice is essential for the GP, who will not only have to insure his life in the event of early death but will also find it necessary to provide cover for more mundane matters such as the house, car and surgery.

For GPs in particular, whose requirements, particularly in the form of pension provision (*see* Chapters 47 and 48) may be very different from most other sections of the community, it is advisable, if not essential, that any insurance adviser consulted understands how GP finance works and therefore can accurately assess a GP's insurance needs.

The Financial Services Act

Introduced in 1986, the purpose of this Act is to give consumers, including investors and policy holders, a measure of legal protection that they have not previously enjoyed.

One feature of the Act is the requirement for those giving advice of a financial and investment nature to be registered under one of the regulatory bodies. Many brokers are registered with FIMBRA (Financial Intermediaries, Managers and Brokers Regulatory Association). Anyone seeking to take out insurance policies or deal with investment matters through such an intermediary or broker should check that the broker is a member of such a regulatory body.

A further feature of the Financial Services Act is that anyone offering such advice must do so honestly and is required, for instance, to offer a policy best equipped to meet the client's needs. For instance, a client should not be advised to take out a policy merely because it pays the broker the highest commission. Indeed, the broker must, on request, disclose to a client the amount of commission he is receiving.

House insurance

A GP will need to insure his private house against such eventualities as fire, burglary and theft. Many insurance companies now offer comprehensive policies including standard cover of this nature.

Fire insurance, in particular, should be kept up to date. A GP should be aware of current property values to ensure that any award is not an underestimate in the event of a loss. The operation of the 'average' clause on insurance claims could mean that, if a householder was under-insured, the insurance company would pay out only an equivalent proportion of the claim. Many insurance companies now offer automatic adjustments to annual building costs so that the cover is maintained at the required level.

Those taking out mortgages to finance private houses will find that such insurance is normally arranged through the building society or other lender, although it is advisable to check that the premiums paid are competitive.

Surgery insurance

Every GP should ensure that full and adequate insurance of the surgery is maintained. Where a surgery is developed (*see* Chapters 27 and 28) and a loan taken out, it is normally a condition of the mortgage that such a policy be maintained on a regular basis. In larger practices, the responsibility for dealing with surgery insurance will generally lie with the practice manager.

A GP should ensure that *all* possible losses are covered by insurance. In certain areas, this may be alleviated by efficient security procedures.

In a group practice, the cost of surgery insurance is normally treated as a partnership expense and is paid by the partners in accordance with their shares of partnership profits.

Car insurance

Virtually all GPs run motor cars and have to insure them, not only for their own protection but in accordance with the law. The insurance of motor cars on anything other than a fully comprehensive basis is not usually beneficial, except in exceptional cases or where the vehicle may not be of significant value.

Some practices are able to make savings in insurance by negotiating a 'group premium' under which all the partners' cars are insured under the same policy. There may be partnership cars used by partners or other staff which are the responsibility of the partnership, and the cost of these should fall on partnership funds.

In a partnership, it is important to establish whether the insurance premiums on the partners' own cars are to be charged against partnership profits or to be met individually by each partner. If, as is normal, the latter arrangement applies, each partner should ensure that the premium is included in his annual claim for car expenses (*see* Chapter 42).

Motor insurance is an extremely competitive market and numerous companies operate in the field. Over the years a few of them have been found to be less than professional in their dealings with policy holders and the motorist should ensure that his insurers are well-established and stable.

Members of the Automobile Association (AA) and other bodies are offered special rates which can be highly competitive. Insuring direct through one of the Lloyds' syndicates can often provide a saving, but in any event the potential insurer is advised to obtain several quotations.

These should be judged on their merits, taking into account not merely the cover provided but the extent to which this is affected by the conditions of no claims bonuses, excess provisions, etc.

Professional insurance (defence societies)

A GP has to insure himself against claims for negligence. Indeed membership of recognized defence societies is normally included in the contracts of hospital doctors and the partnership deeds of GPs. It is also a condition of acceptance onto the list of an FHSA, and by the local medical committee.

Reduced rates normally apply to GPs in the early stages of their careers and to some retired doctors.

Public liability policies

All practices should have, probably as part of a normal comprehensive cover, an insurance against claims by patients and others, possibly including members of staff, for injuries incurred in or around the surgery which could be held to be due to the negligence of the GP or practice. Although such a policy may form part of a larger package, a GP should ensure that cover of this type is in place.

Loss of profits insurance

Such a policy covers any loss of income that may arise from a fire or similar occurrence. Again, this is often built into a comprehensive package.

Permanent health (locum) insurance

The GP will need cover in the event of being unable to work through illness or injury. Such cover is referred to as permanent health insurance, although in the medical profession it is frequently termed 'locum insurance' because the effect of the claim on the policy will be to pay locums in the absence of the GP from normal duties.

This is a specialized market and the GP should seek advice from brokers with expertise in offering insurance advice to the medical profession.

No tax relief is allowed in respect of premiums paid by GPs for their own cover. Policies are arranged so that the benefit is received free of tax for a complete fiscal year.

However, schemes set up for the benefit of practice staff are tax deductible to the partnership or employer, and will not attract extra National Insurance contributions from either the employer or employee. However, the benefit is payable to the employer and is treated as a receipt of the business for tax purposes. This is then offset when passed on to the employee as a continuation of salary. The income benefit the employee receives will be taxed under PAYE and will be subject to normal National Insurance deductions.

Medical insurance

Some GPs may wish to insure the cost of private medical treatment should they or their families fall ill. This is frequently done through such organizations as BUPA or the Private Patients' Plan. Substantial discounts can be obtained if a group scheme is in operation.

Family income benefit

The NHS Pension Scheme (Chapter 47) provides relatively low benefit in the event of the death of a younger practitioner in service. A young GP is advised, therefore, to take out a policy that covers his family and will provide a continuing level of income in the event of an early death. It is sensible to provide cover, at least while any children are undergoing full-time education. It may also be advisable for a male GP to insure his wife; if she were to die and it became necessary to employ a nurse or housekeeper, the cost would be significant. Such cover is not unduly expensive and would provide the main protection against the financial effects of an unexpected bereavement.

Life insurance

It is advisable for a GP to have personal life cover in addition to that provided by the NHSPS, particularly in the early years when financial commitments to the family are at their most demanding, and death benefits under the NHSPS are providing only a low level of protection.

There has been no tax relief available on new life assurance policies since 1984, except for those who are eligible to make contributions to a personal pension plan; for example, those GPs who have earnings from private consultancy work or NHS earnings in excess of their superannuable income.

Some mortgage protection policies also qualify for tax relief under personal pension plan legislation, but there are special limits and Inland Revenue restrictions on both term assurance and mortgage protection premiums. Expert advice is, therefore, essential.

Critical illness protection

Most medical and hospital personnel can now provide cover for themselves and their families against HIV infection contracted as a result of an accident during normal occupational duties, as well as a comprehenisve range of other conditions, such as heart attack, cancer, paralysis and total disability. This is provided by a limited number of insurance companies only and is certainly not available on all critical illness plans.

School fees

For those families proposing to educate children privately, a popular means of financing this is through prior investment in life assurance policies specially tailored for that purpose.

However, for those who have left it too late to use a qualifying policy, which will normally have a minimum term of 10 years before maturity, other options are now available.

One of the most popular methods of funding for school fees now is by investing in personal equity plans (PEPs). These are both tax efficient and flexible, in that they offer tax-free growth, and can be surrendered at any time. There are, however, some drawbacks in using this type of investment.

Firstly, PEPs offer a greater degree of risk, in that their value can fall as well as rise, and secondly they do not offer any form of life cover, which would therefore have to be taken out separately.

A more innovative development by one or two banks and building societies has been the introduction of a 'draw-down' facility. This involves a re-mortgage to include the additional loan required to pay the total amount of school fees, together with a cheque book facility to pay the fees as and when required.

The interest payable on the total loan is at normal mortgage lending rates, and is only payable on the additional part of the loan as and when the fees are required. The loan can be repaid at the end of the mortgage term, either by the tax-free cash available under the NHSPS, with the lost pension benefit replaced by a free-standing additional voluntary contribution plan (FSAVC), or alternatively by some other savings plan.

Tax relief

Most of the premiums deriving from the types of policy set out above will be at least partially allowable for income tax purposes. It is important, however, to understand exactly how and to what extent this will be granted.

Surgery insurance

Premiums on such policies are normally included as an item of practice expense in the annual accounts, and the tax relief will be granted fully as a regular item of expenditure. This will apply to fire, burglary, public liability, loss of profits and similar insurances.

Private houses

Those GPs who are able to sustain a claim for a proportion of their house expenses (*see* page 244) are normally able to include premiums on house insurance policies in such a claim and receive in effect such a proportion of the relief as has been agreed with the Inland Revenue.

Motor insurance

Similarly, all premiums on motor cars used wholly or partly for practice purposes should be included in an overall claim for car expenses (*see* Chapter 42), but will be subject to a restriction for private use agreed with the Inland Revenue.

Employers' liability insurance

All GPs employing staff should ensure they are covered for possible claims from staff members who may suffer injury or loss whilst at work, and may subsequently be able to show that their employer has been negligent. Such premiums are normally fully allowable for tax purposes.

47 Superannuation and Pensions

MANY GPs take an active interest in planning for retirement only in the years immediately approaching that date. This is unfortunate because the effect of any change is limited by the number of years during which benefits can accrue. A GP who plans for retirement in his early thirties is far wiser than the GP who does so in his mid-fifties. All GPs should keep their pension facilities, and the opportunity they bring, under constant review—circumstances change during a GP's working life and so needs vary; in the same way, legislation and changes in procedure determine the various arrangements available from time to time.

The NHS Pension Scheme (NHSPS)

The present superannuation scheme dates back to the formation of the NHS in 1948. Fundamentally the scheme has remained unaltered, although there have been a number of radical and far-reaching amendments. Some of these have come into force only during the last two or three years, and in many cases GPs and their advisers are not yet fully aware of their implications.

The NHSPS is divided in effect into two separate schemes. One for general practitioners (ie medical, dental and ophthalmic contractors to the NHS) is based on 'dynamized' career earnings; the total earnings of the practitioner during his career are taken into account in arriving at the final pension and lump sum entitlement. The other scheme applies to officers, ie doctors, dentists and others employed in hospitals or other NHS services on a salaried basis. The ultimate benefits from this scheme are calculated on a 'final salary' basis which is outside the scope of this book.

It is not possible to explore all aspects of the NHSPS in a book of this size, but this chapter and the following one give an outline of the scheme, the range of benefits offered to GPs and the additional facilities available. In conclusion, further sources are specified from which the reader can obtain additional information.

Superannuable income

Superannuable income consists of all earnings of the GP as a contractor to the NHS, less an annually agreed average deduction for notional expenses. Currently, this estimated expenses element (calculated annually) is 35.5%.

There are, however, exceptions to this. Whilst that figure is deducted from all standard items of earning, such as capitation fees, BPA, item of service fees, etc, certain other items of income, such as the seniority allowance, training grant and target payments are fully superannuable, ie without making the standard deduction for expenses.

Some items are not superannuable. These include refunds, eg of practice staff costs and rates, and reimbursements such as the notional and cost rent allowances. A list of fees and allowances that are wholly, partly or non-superannuable is shown in Box 47.1.

Box 47.1: The NHS superannuation scheme—superannuable income

Fully superannuable (100%)

- Seniority allowance.
- Training grant.
- Course organizer training grant.
- Target payments
- Designated area allowance
- Inducement payments
- Transitional payments
- Hospital appointments (clinical assistantships, hospital practitioners, clinics, locums, staff funds).

Partly superannuable (67.5%)

- Basic practice allowance.
- Assistant allowance.
- Capitation fees.
- Deprivation payments.
- Maternity medical service fees.
- Contraceptive service fees.
- Temporary resident, immediately necessary treatment, emergency treatment, dental haemorrhage arrest and anaesthetic fees.
- Night visit fees.
- Capitation addition for out-of-hours cover.
- Initial practice allowance.
- Rural practice payments.
- Dispensing fees, on-cost, oxygen therapy service rents and fees.
- Postgraduate education allowance.
- Students allowance.
- Registration fees.
- Health promotion payments.
- Child health surveillance fees.
- Minor surgery sessional fees.

Box 47.1: *continued.*

Non-superannuable
- Non-NHS fees:
    private patients
    insurance medicals
    sundry fees: cremations, private certificates, etc.
- Notional and cost rent allowances.
- Sickness and maternity payments.
- Prolonged study leave locum payments.
- Locum payments for single-handed rural GPs attending courses.
- Reimbursements; rent and rates; practice staff; computing costs; trainees' salaries.
- Associate allowance.
- Doctors retainer scheme allowance.
- Net ingredient cost, container allowance and VAT paid in respect of supply of drugs and appliances.
- Trainee car allowance and other trainees' expenses.
- Fundholding management allowance.

A typical calculation of annual superannuation contributions is set out in Figure 47.1, although, in practice, this is calculated quarterly throughout the year.

Dr A has gross income for 1993/94 from NHS fees and allowances of £40 000, with a Stage III seniority award of £5955. He is a GP trainer and receives the training grant of £3870.

His superannuation contribution is calculated thus:

	£	£
Fees and allowances	40 000	
Less: Notional expenses (35.5%)	14 200	
		25 800
Seniority	5955	
Training grant	3870	
		9825
		35 625
Contribution at 6%		2138

Figure 47.1 Calculation of superannuation contributions

Method of contribution

Contributions by each GP are calculated by the FHSA and shown as deductions on each quarterly remittance statement. It is important, particularly in partnerships where there are differing shares, or where some partners are making additional contributions, that these deductions are reflected in drawings paid to the GPs, either monthly or quarterly.

GPs in partnership

For GPs in partnership, their contributions are calculated by the FHSA according to the profit-sharing ratios in force. It is important for partnerships to give their FHSAs full notification of each change in profit-sharing ratios at regular intervals so that these can be reflected in their superannuation deductions. Failure to do so can result in partners suffering in terms of their ultimate pension entitlement.

Contribution levels

At present, GPs who belong to the scheme contribute 6% of the NHS superannuable remuneration to the NHSPS.

In addition, the NHS makes an annual payment of 4% of superannuable remuneration for these GPs.

Contributions and tax relief

Unlike the statutory tax relief granted on contributions to the NHSPS for those in the salaried sector, that available to GPs is concessionary. It is provided by Extra-Statutory Concession A9, and must be claimed by GPs each year.

It is important that, when the annual accounts are drawn up, the contributions are shown separately in the current accounts of each partner, rather than being shown as a deduction in calculating the partnership profits. This is in order to receive tax relief on the contributions to both the basic and any additional schemes on an actual year rather than a preceding year basis. There is a time benefit in the tax relief being granted in this way.

Tax relief on these contributions should be claimed on the GP's personal income tax return and not by inclusion in the practice accounts or in a separate claim for personal practice expenses.

Benefits of the scheme

The benefits available to GPs who are members of the NHSPS are several and substantially more than a pension and lump sum entitlement.

1 A pension which is index-linked and is calculated upon 1.4% of the uprated (dynamized) career earnings of the GP concerned.
2 A lump sum retiring allowance, entirely free of tax, normally 4.2% of the uprated career earnings (or three times the annual pension). The lump sum will not, however, reach that figure if the GP was a married man in practice before 1972, and who has not bought the unreduced lump sum.
3 Widow's and, in appropriate cases, widower's pension.
4 Children's benefit for the GP whose career is terminated by death.
5 A death gratuity.
6 Ill-health retirement benefits if a GP is obliged to cease work through illness after two or more years' service.

The NHSPS offers an attractive package for GPs, particularly for those who have younger dependants. However, these benefits can be relatively modest during the earlier years of service and the younger GP may find it prudent to take out some form of family income benefit assurance to ensure a continuing and satisfactory level of income for any surviving family (see page 273).

Opting out of the scheme

Since 1988, GPs have been entitled to opt out of the NHSPS. However, it is doubtful that such a course of action would be of benefit to the GP concerned. A GP contemplating this course should bear in mind the implication of relinquishing a series of valuable rights, which would be difficult and expensive to buy in the private sector, most notably the indexation of the pension, the cost of which would be enormous on the open market.

The 'dynamizing' factor

The pension of a practitioner is calculated by reference to total career superannuable earnings. These will include amounts earned during the early part of a GP's career, almost certainly at much lower levels of income than those in force at the time of retirement. If no adjustment is made, a pension calculation based on these figures would produce benefits much lower than those enjoyed by an employed doctor, whose pension is based upon a 'final salary' calculation.

To overcome this disadvantage, the principle of uprating or 'dynamizing' was formulated, by which a factor agreed and updated each year is applied to the superannuable remuneration for each year in order to convert the amount of income in the year in which it was earned to its equivalent value at the date of retirement. Those factors currently in force are shown in Table 47.1.

Table 47.1 Calculation of dynamizing factors (applied to GPs' superannuable pay to calculate final pension entitlement)

Year ending March 31	Dynamizing factor	Year ending March 31	Dynamizing factor
1949	24.032	1971	8.346
1950	24.032	1972	7.727
1951	22.232	1973	7.186
1952	22.232	1974	6.967
1953	22.232	1975	6.373
1954	22.232	1976	4.586
1955	22.232	1977	4.470
1956	22.232	1978	4.302
1957	22.121	1979	3.298
1958	20.081	1980	2.805
1959	19.803	1981	2.363
1960	18.933	1982	2.229
1961	18.103	1983	2.110
1962	18.103	1984	1.975
1963	18.103	1985	1.853
1964	15.879	1986	1.726
1965	15.879	1987	1.624
1966	14.437	1988	1.493
1967	13.417	1989	1.391
1968	10.828	1990	1.288
1969	10.612	1991	1.191
1970	10.016	1992	1.068

The table lists dynamizing factors that GPs can use to calculate their pension if it became payable on 31 March 1991. If they retired after 31 March 1989, it can be used to obtain an estimate of benefits and be brought up to date when the table is superseded. GPs can get a copy of their computerized superannuable pay record from the NHS pension funds office.

It is these uprated or dynamized figures that are aggregated and upon which the calculation for final retirement benefit is based (*see* Figure 47.2).

Dr X, who has practised in the NHS since 1955, retired on 30 September 1990, having purchased additional years to bring his service up to 40 years, as well as the unreduced lump sum.

His total career NHS earnings were £500 000 which, after the operation of the dynamizing factor, gives uprated career earnings of £1 200 000.

He will receive an annual pension of 1.4% of that amount, ie £16 800 per annum, together with a lump sum entitlement of 4.2%, or £50 400.

Figure 47.2   Calculation of final retirement benefits

Hospital service

Most GPs, at some time, will have worked in the hospital service—usually before embarking upon general practice but also perhaps as a clinical assistant in the hospital practitioner service—or have received some form of salary from the NHS in addition to their GP income. This salary is fully superannuable; therefore GPs may accrue an additional pension based upon this.

To take account of this other service, depending on its length, a GP will receive either a pro rata increase of the practitioner pension or an additional officer pension in respect of hospital service. In addition, a lump sum is received which can be up to three times the annual pension.

It should be noted that where practitioners have hospital appointments of this nature, they may stay in the NHSPS in respect of their 'practitioner' service, but opt out of it with regard to their hospital posts.

Purchase of additional benefits

The Inland Revenue does not allow total superannuable service to exceed 45 years, of which not more than 40 may accrue before the age of 60 years.

As most practitioners qualify at about the age of 24 years, it is not possible for more than 36 years of superannuable service to be acquired by the age of 60; in many cases, it will be less and a GP would be unable to retire on what is seen to be a full pension. For this reason, facilities have been introduced within the NHSPS for the purchase of additional service in the form of 'added years'.

The added years scheme

The present scheme for purchase of added years was introduced in the early 1980s. Its main feature is that the practitioner contracts to pay a fixed additional proportion of NHS superannuable earnings into the scheme for which extra benefits will be received, in the form of pension and lump sum on retirement.

There are two limitations.

1 Total service worked and added years purchased must not exceed 40 years at age 60.
2 The maximum permitted contribution to the scheme is 15% of the super- annuable remuneration, including the standard 6%, so that the maximum allowed payment for added years cannot exceed 9% of that remuneration.

For younger practitioners, the cost of buying their full entitlement will be considerably less than 9%, but for those of more senior years the effect of the 9% limit is likely to mean that they are unable to purchase all the added years for which they are eligible. Current calculations, in percentage terms, for purchasing these added years are shown in Table 47.2 (1).

The unreduced lump sum

Married male practitioners in the NHS before March 1972 will receive a lump sum retiring allowance for each year of service prior to that date at one-third of the rate applicable to each year subsequent to March 1972. However, a facility is available that enables such GPs to purchase the missing proportion of their lump sum. The principles and limitations of the scheme are similar to those for buying added years and the costs of this are also set out in Table 47.2 (2).

Contributions to private schemes

GPs in the NHS, both doctors and dentists, are in a unique position in that, whilst self-employed, they are also members of an occupational pension scheme. This unusual status provides them with opportunities not always available to other self-employed people, which enable them to make private pension provision in respect of:

1 non-superannuable income ('topping-up')
2 superannuable earnings, if tax relief on contributions to the NHSPS is renounced
3 earnings of a spouse employed by a practitioner or his practice (this is discussed more fully in Chapter 43).

Table 47.2   Additional NHS benefits

1   Cost of buying added years (fixed percentage to nominated birthday)

Extra % of pay required as additional contributions to buy one year of additional service—when paid from the 'Age next birthday' to the 'Chosen birthday'

| Age next birthday | Chosen birthday | | Age next birthday | Chosen birthday | | Age next birthday | Chosen birthday | |
	60	65		60	65		60	65
	%	%		%	%		%	%
20	0.50	0.36	35	0.85	0.67	50	2.25	1.38
21	0.52	0.38	36	0.89	0.69	51	2.53	1.48
22	0.54	0.40	37	0.93	0.72	52	2.86	1.60
23	0.56	0.42	38	0.98	0.74	53	3.26	1.74
24	0.58	0.44	39	1.03	0.77	54	3.80	1.90
25	0.60	0.46	40	1.09	0.80	55	4.58	2.08
26	0.62	0.48	41	1.15	0.83	56	5.77	2.30
27	0.64	0.50	42	1.22	0.87	57	7.77	2.56
28	0.66	0.52	43	1.30	0.91	58	12.06	2.92
29	0.68	0.54	44	1.39	0.95	59	–	3.40
30	0.70	0.56	45	1.48	1.00	60	–	4.10
31	0.72	0.58	46	1.58	1.06	61	–	5.20
32	0.75	0.60	47	1.70	1.13	62	–	6.97
33	0.78	0.62	48	1.85	1.21	63	–	10.42
34	0.81	0.64	49	2.03	1.29			

2   Cost of purchasing the unreduced lump sum (GPs practising before 1972 as married men)

Extra % of pay required as additional contributions to buy a bigger lump sum for one year—when paid from 'Age next birthday' to the 'Chosen birthday'

| Age next birthday | Chosen birthday | | Age next birthday | Chosen birthday | | Age next birthday | Chosen birthday | |
	60	65		60	65		60	65
	%	%		%	%		%	%
30	0.08	0.07	41	0.13	0.10	53	0.38	0.20
31	0.08	0.07	42	0.14	0.10	54	0.45	0.22
32	0.09	0.07	43	0.15	0.11	55	0.54	0.24
33	0.09	0.07	44	0.16	0.11	56	0.68	0.27
34	0.10	0.08	45	0.17	0.12	57	0.91	0.30
35	0.10	0.08	46	0.19	0.12	58	1.42	0.34
36	0.11	0.08	47	0.20	0.13	59	–	0.40
37	0.11	0.08	48	0.22	0.14	60	–	0.48
38	0.12	0.09	49	0.24	0.15	61	–	0.61
39	0.12	0.09	50	0.27	0.16	62	–	0.82
40	0.13	0.09	51	0.30	0.17	63	–	1.23
			52	0.34	0.19			

'Topping-up'

A GP has the facility to pay private pension contributions on the proportion of relevant earnings, ie Schedule D taxable income, derived from non-NHS sources. This process is popularly known as 'topping-up' and is calculated by multiplying the standard contribution to the NHSPS in any given year by a factor of 100/6, such product then being compared with the Schedule D income. If the Schedule D income is higher, contributions can be made to a private scheme. The method of calculation is shown in Figure 47.3.

In practice, most GPs, with little or no income from outside the NHS, are unlikely to be in a position to benefit from this.

The calculation must take into account the GP's Schedule D medical earnings from all sources, not merely those from GP partnership.

Those with non-NHS earnings should make a provision for them in order to gain tax advantages and a higher total income in retirement.

Dr A, a GP aged 47 years, who in 1993/94 had income assessable to Schedule D tax amounting to £35 000, is considering paying retirement annuity premiums. During the year ended 5 April 1994 he paid total superannuation contributions to the FHSA amounting to £2950, including added years and unreduced lump sum payments of £1050.

	£
Superannuation paid: 1993/94	2950
Less: Added years and unreduced lump sum payments	1050
	1900
Grossed-up: £1900 × 100/6 =	31 667
Schedule D income	35 000
Non-superannuable income	3333
Allowable pension premiums: 17.5%	583

Dr A therefore can pay only £583 by way of private pension premiums upon which he will obtain tax relief at his highest rate.

Figure 47.3 'Topping-up': calculation

Renunciation of tax relief

Relief may also be relinquished. In such circumstances, a GP may make private pension provisions for earnings already superannuated under the NHSPS. This reduces tax relief on the payment for the private pension by the amount of relief not claimed on contributions to the NHSPS. This is an extremely valuable option and one that should be exploited whenever possible. However, such a procedure involves any GP in a much greater outgoing from his disposable income and he must be satisfied that such expenditure will not cause undue financial difficulty. A typical calculation is shown in Figure 47.4.

Dr B is a GP aged 58 years with NHS superannuable remuneration for 1993/94 of £35 000 and a Schedule D tax assessment of £31 500. His top rate of tax is 40%. His contribution to the NHSPS is 6% of £35 000, or £2100 per annum. If tax relief at 40% is claimed on this, his net expenditure is £1260.

Dr B decides to remain in the NHSPS but not to claim relief on his contributions and pay the maximum permitted amount to a private pension policy. His net outlay will now be:

		£
NHSPS contribution 6% of £35 000		2100
Private premium (maximum) 35% of £31 500		11 025
		13 125
Tax relief 40% of £11 025		4410
	Total net cost	8715

So, whilst the exercise results in more tax relief being available to Dr B, this is not the most significant feature. By making these arrangements, his net outlay has risen from £1260 to £8715, by which means he has purchased additional pension benefit.

However good the potential benefits from the scheme, it is vital that the cost of their acquisition is appreciated.

Figure 47.4   Renunciation of tax relief calculation

A GP's decision to renounce tax relief on NHS contributions is an annual election, ie a GP can decide each year whether or not to pursue this course. Such an election can be made for the present year of assessment and the preceding tax year. Beyond that, retrospective renunciation is possible only for those years on which assessable income has not been finalized.

Free-standing additional voluntary contributions (FSAVCs)

FSAVCs give practitioners a private sector alternative to the public sector added years scheme. They are available through various life offices and other pension providers. FSAVCs provide pension only without any lump sum.

At some time, a practitioner is likely to be asked to decide between buying added years or FSAVCs, and he should be aware of the advantages and disadvantages of each, which are set out in Box 47.2.

The limit for contributions is the same as that for added years, ie a GP buying standard contributions at 6% can contribute only another 9% to the FSAVC scheme. There is a further limitation in that GPs who have already acquired—including added years purchased—entitlement to 39.1 years of pension entitlement will be unable to contribute to the FSAVC scheme.

Basic rate tax relief on FSAVCs is allowed by deduction at source. GPs who are in the higher tax bracket will obtain additional relief through their normal income tax assessments.

These, then, are the prime means by which a GP can provide for an adequate income during retirement.

Box 47.2: FSAVCs versus added years

Advantages of FSAVCs over added years

1 Greater flexibility with the option of irregular payments.
2 Added years, once started, are difficult to drop unless extreme financial hardship can be proved.
3 Added years can be prohibitively expensive for older GPs.
4 Tax relief at standard rate obtained at source.
5 Provide a 'mix' of public sector basic benefits and private sector additional benefits.

Advantages of added years over FSAVCs

1 No facility to buy tax-free lump sum with FSAVCs.
2 Added years are index-linked.
3 FSAVCs offer no protection in enforced early retirement through ill-health.
4 No ancillary benefits unless acquired separately.
5 The possibility of the FSAVC scheme being overfunded. This may occur if the possible benefit is in excess of 66% of final remuneration and could lead to taxation of the pension fund on retirement.
6 Added years do not depend on the investment performance of the pension fund.

48 Retirement

FOR those approaching retirement, the prospect can be a source of considerable anxiety. Can the accustomed lifestyle of GPs be maintained on a post-retirement income? Some practitioners may be unduly pessimistic as a result of an inaccurate and/or incomplete interpretation of the inevitable financial changes that retirement produces. Unless these are identified and appreciated, a highly misleading impression of finances in retirement can result.

The three changes of greatest significance are:

1 reduction in income
2 increase in capital
3 loss of Schedule D tax status.

Let us now look at these separately.

1 Reduction in income

The income reduction is often less than the GP has envisaged. This is because practitioners frequently make pointless comparisons between their NHS pension and the gross earnings it replaces. The NHS pension is taxable income and it should be related to its taxed, not gross, pre-retirement equivalent.

Another factor often ignored is the yield from investment of the NHS lump sum retirement allowance. In many instances practitioners also have some non-superannuable NHS income and earnings from private patient and/or outside sources. The latter may be from an outside appointment, insurance medicals or writing and/or tutoring. Private pension provisions in respect of the taxable income from such sources is permitted and prudent GPs should make sure that appropriate pension arrangements are made for any such income. There are significant tax benefits to be gained from private pensions, which can limit the reduction in income on retirement.

2 Increase in capital

In addition to the tax-free NHSPS lump sum and/or private pension received at retirement, many GPs will have 'new' capital arising, for example, from the sale of their share of practice premises, and the receipt of the proceeds from assurance policies, saving schemes and other investments tailored to terminate at retirement. If the yield from investment of these capital sums is taken into account, the earnings/pension gap can be significantly less than anticipated. It is vital that such capital is wisely invested, in order to counter-act other factors, described below.

3 Loss of Schedule D tax status

This can have adverse implications for a retired GP. During the GP's working life, tax relief will have been obtained on certain items of annual expenditure; not all such outlay stops with retirement, but the tax saving in respect of it will cease. The extent to which this affects individual GPs varies according to their particular circumstances, but the disadvantage can be considerable.

Index-linked pensions

Working GPs have many opportunities to increase their current earnings, but once they have retired nothing can be done to alter or influence the pension payable to them.

However, index linking, offered by NHS, National Insurance and some private pensions, provides extra money each year. Whilst it does not represent a rise in real terms, index linking protects the purchasing potential of pensions. For the majority, the only real rises in retirement income will be those resulting from the adoption of a suitable investment strategy.

The lump sum

In addition to a pension, GPs receive a tax-free lump sum as part of their retirement benefit from the NHSPS. For practitioners with no NHS service before March 1972, the lump sum will be three times the initial pension. For married men with pre-March 1972 service, who have not purchased the unreduced lump sum, it will equal their pension for the years prior to March 1972 and be three times their subsequent pension. Married female practi-tioners, who elect to purchase a widower's pension based on their service before April 1988, will have their lump sum reduced for service during that period. However, it is possible for such a shortfall to be purchased.

It is vital for GPs to remember that their lump sum is the commuted value of part of their pension. The attraction is that, had that money been paid as a pension, it would have been taxable. The lump sum is free of tax, although the yield from its investment may or may not be taxable, depending upon the sources selected. Moreover, a GP can, of course, benefit from the lump sum immediately, which may be desirable if he or she does not expect to live long.

Many GPs feel that their lump sum should be deposited to produce optimum instant interest or used to reduce or repay a debt. Frequently, however, neither of these courses is desirable, and it is essential that all the financial circumstances, past and future, are taken into account when the deployment of retirement capital is being contemplated.

Retirement age

GPs may only receive normal retirement benefits from the NHSPS on or after the age of 60 years, except in cases of early retirement on grounds of ill health. At present, benefits can accrue up to age 65 years or until 45 years of superannuable service have elapsed. It may be possible to extend pensionable age beyond age 65, but not past 70-years-old. Whether it is prudent for any NHS service after age 65 to be superannuable will depend on the personal circumstances of the GP.

Date of retirement

A GP should not normally retire at the end of a month as the method of calculation for retirement benefits gives a slight advantage if retirement is deferred until a few days into the following month.

24-hour retirement

At 60-years-old, a GP may take normal retirement benefits and, a day later, return to practice. Provided the pension plus subsequent NHS superannuable earnings do not together amount to more than the average pre-retirement earnings, then the pension is paid in full. Should the two produce a sum greater than the defined average, then the pension is 'abated' (ie reduced) by the amount of the excess. There are two immediate advantages from this procedure.

1 There is little difference between total income received following a 24-hour retirement and that received prior to the partial retirement from a larger share of NHS income, despite the fact that fewer hours are usually worked.
2 The receipt of the tax free lump sum retiring allowance.

If a 24-hour retirement is taken between the ages of 60 and 65, subsequent earnings can be superannuated under the NHSPS. Although such income is likely to be lower following 24-hour retirement, to avoid or minimize abatement of pension, a GP's pension in full retirement may not be significantly less than if the 24-hour retirement had not been taken. Indeed, if certain steps are taken following a 24-hour retirement, it may be possible for the GP's overall retirement income to be greater than if he had not partially retired. The 24-hour retirement may also benefit the other members of the partnership.

GPs contemplating 24-hour retirement should seek specialist guidance, as the figures may easily be misinterpreted. It is important to bear in mind that only the NHS superannuable remuneration received subsequent to a 24-hour retirement is relevant when the abatement calculation is made. Other earnings, irrespective of their source or amount, are irrelevant in this context.

The lump sum obtained with 24-hour retirement

Some of the decisions regarding the investment of a lump sum are of particular relevance to a GP who takes a 24-hour retirement.

As has already been stated, there is unlikely to be much difference between the total incomes of a practitioner pre- and post-24-hour retirement. Thus it may be counterproductive to invest the lump sum to provide immediate income which may be surplus to requirement, as this may be wholly taxable and its receipt could be at the expense of a higher income in total retirement. If the lump sum obtained with 24-hour retirement is used to generate extra income immediately, this will exacerbate the drop in total income that occurs with full retirement. The prime investment objective of most GPs should, on the contrary, be to reduce that drop in income. Tax efficient opportunities exist for practitioners, in this context, which should be urgently and profitably pursued.

Post-retirement earnings

Some GPs choose to continue working after retirement, as locums, for government departments, or as medical advisers to commercial organizations. Income from these sources is taxable, and the GP is responsible for returning details of earnings to the Inland Revenue.

Provided a GP has reached the age of 65 years for men or 60 for women, he or she is not liable for any National Insurance contributions arising from these earnings. However, private pension contributions can be refunded on any agreed taxable profit. Such earnings, provided they are not derived from an NHS superannuable source, do not count towards the abatement of a GP's pension. However, contributions to a private pension can and should be made in respect of the taxable income from such earnings.

A retired GP is likely to require additional advice on various aspects of taxation and financial and estate planning. All these subjects can be discussed at length with a professional adviser and steps taken to obtain the maximum advantage available.

Further advice and reading

Any GP who is a member of the BMA will be able to obtain advice from the BMA on all aspects of his or her pension.

A GP wishing to obtain separate advice can contact the Medical and Dental Retirement Advisory Service (MADRAS), Hertlands House, Primett Road, Stevenage, Herts SG1 3EE (telephone 0438 742727). MADRAS is a society funded by members' subscriptions, which publishes a regular series of reports and updates on all aspects of pensions legislation affecting GPs.

A booklet called *Signpost 5*, written by John Dean with Douglas Shields of MADRAS, was published in late 1988 by the Bureau of Medical Practitioner Affairs, Rigby Hall, Rigby Lane, Bromsgrove, Worcestershire B60 2EW (telephone 021 525 8706), and is the most up-to-date and complete work currently available on the subject of pensions and retirement for GPs.

49 The GP and his Accountant

ALTHOUGH the average GP will come across many professional advisers during his working life, it will probably be the accountant who is his most regular professional adviser. A GP relies on his accountant to keep the finances of the practice and family in good order. It is a relationship that can and should be extremely rewarding on both sides, with the accountant accepted as a trusted and confidential adviser over the years, ready to offer advice at short notice. Yet the opposite is frequently the case, with the GP feeling that he is not being particularly well served. Some practices may engage four or five different firms of accountants in not many more years. Indeed, many practices may question whether they need an accountant at all.

Is an accountant necessary?

In theory, no; in practice, probably yes. A GP can negotiate taxation with the Inland Revenue and prepare his own accounts for submission and for agreement by the partners. Occasionally, single-handed practitioners may prepare their own accounts. However, in an average practice, particularly the larger partnership, the average GP has not the necessary professional skills to prepare accounts that preserve equity among the partners. Indeed, it is debatable whether any GP, after his surgical duties have been completed, would be willing and able to devote the necessary time and skill to the accounts.

Moreover, the partnership deed may contain a clause requiring the accounts to be prepared by a named qualified accountant. It is difficult justify the removal of such a clause. The advent of fundholding (*see* Chapter 34) further enhances the role of the practice accountant. Indeed fundholding accounts should be prepared by a specialist in the field.

An accountant's duties

The basic duties of the accountant are to prepare the annual practice accounts and agree these with the Inland Revenue. He will also recommend payments of tax, submit computations for agreement and deal with allocations of tax payments and repayments. These are sometimes referred to as 'compliance' matters, since they largely represent legal requirements which must be complied with. In many practices, the accountant will also be called upon to advise on a range of peripheral matters, such as drawings calculations, tax reserves, surgery developments, pensions and retirement, and provision of management information.

If invited to act for any GPs individually, an accountant will deal with their personal tax returns and expenses claims, as well as advising on other aspects of their personal finances.

Judging an accountant's competence

Is he doing his job properly, and how can we tell if that is the case?

It is notoriously difficult for one professional to judge the competence of another. However, it is possible to lay down a few general rules by which a GP can form an opinion as to whether the accountant is doing a good job.

1 Are the accounts delivered within a reasonable time after each year-end? If not, it may be the result of lack of information being given to the accountant; if it can be established that the accountant is at fault, he should be made to understand that much of the value of accounts of this nature lies in their prompt production and delivery.

2 Do the accounts give an idea of the manner in which income is generated and expenses paid? Do they show exactly how the profits are allocated among the partners and do they give the level of management information that will enable the practice to be run economically and efficiently? A specimen set of such accounts is shown in Chapter 18, whilst Chapter 19 interprets statistics which can be extracted from these.

3 Is he a specialist? Does he have a copy of the Red Book available for easy reference and can he discuss with you aspects of finance exclusive to GPs, such as pensions and superannuation, cost rent schemes, practice allowances, leave advances and item of service fees?

It is now possible for accountants to purchase the Red Book, so all accountants presuming to act for doctors should possess a copy.

4 Is he efficient? Are letters answered reasonably promptly and are telephone calls returned?

The specialist accountant

Considerable benefits can be gained by a GP who engages an accountant with experience in dealing with several similar practices and who has made work for GPs his speciality. As this is crucial to the quality of service offered, any GP or practice wishing to engage an accountant should seek to confirm that a prospective accountant is a specialist. Frequently, this can be done only by personal recommendation.

Fees

The judging and evaluation of accountancy fees is probably one of the most misunderstood aspects of the accountant's function. Such fees tend to increase at a steady rate, mainly due to the competitive salaries required within the accountancy profession. These increases may at times be in excess of the rate of inflation.

All accountants charge fees by means of an hourly rate which is applied to the number of hours spent on each particular client's work, with regard to the seniority of the person involved. It is incumbent upon an accountant to employ on each client's affairs the least expensive person possible without any loss of efficiency. For instance, the routine work of agreeing and balancing a petty cash book can be performed by a junior clerk.

However, the rates applied vary not only within an accountancy firm, but between different firms and in different parts of the country. In general higher rates are applied in the South East than in the North of England or Scotland.

The vogue for judging fee levels at a fixed charge per partner for a practice should be discouraged. This is inequitable and frequently not precisely defined, in that such quotations rarely set out whether the fee includes that for the partner's personal work and for VAT. In addition, it presupposes that the cost of dealing with an eight-doctor partnership will be twice that of dealing with a four-doctor practice. This is highly unlikely; the cost may be rather higher, but certainly not double. Indeed, there is a substantial economy of scale in dealing with the larger partnerships. The cost per partner tends to reduce significantly with the number of GPs in a particular practice.

Accountancy fees vary according to numerous factors that cannot always be foreseen: the quality of records given to the accountant; the frequency of partnership changes; whether there are Inland Revenue enquiries into the practice tax affairs; the level of personal work required by individual partners, and other matters. Having said that, the accountancy fees charged for a medium to large partnership (say, from four to seven partners) should not normally exceed 2% of the gross practice income. If so, the practice would probably be justified in asking for an explanation. If the fees are below 1% in a non-dispensing practice, it may be questionable whether sufficiently qualified staff are engaged upon the accounts.

Personal or partnership accountant?

In partnerships, confusion often arises over whether partners should engage the same accountant who deals with practice affairs to deal with their personal finances.

If a GP has confidence in the partnership accountant, there are many advantages in using the same firm—there should be savings of costs due to minimizing correspondence and telephone calls and a single accountant can obtain an overview of the practice affairs which might not otherwise be possible.

Small or large firm?

One decision the doctor will have to make on engaging an accountant is whether he wishes to use a small or large accountancy firm. There are advantages associated with both and it is important that these are appreciated.

Although the small firm may offer a less expensive and more personal service, it may not offer the level of speciality a GP requires and problems can arise when partners/principals retire or are away through periods of holiday or sickness.

A large firm will probably be able to offer a degree of speciality and the accounts will be constantly reviewed by several individuals before the work is completed. This process of review and checking so common in larger firms may increase the fees but it is in a client's interests. However, a GP may feel that in a larger firm his individual requirements are not always catered for and that a less personal service is provided.

Ultimately, it is for each GP to decide. Before making a final decision he should interview various firms. It is worth remembering that, apart from the normal professional duties, an accountant offers peace of mind, and a GP can feel secure in the knowledge that his finances are in good hands and there is no cause for worry when letters, assessment notices and the like arrive from the Inland Revenue.

50 The Practice Banker

> 'Like many other beings, a banker is easier to recognize than to define.'
>
> *Lord Denning*

PERHAPS of more use is a definition given in 1871 by JW Gilbart that 'the exchanging of money; the lending of money; the borrowing of money; the transmitting of money are the four principal branches of the business of modern banking'. This definition recognizes the facts for we are told that Sir Thomas Gresham was the Goldsmiths' banker in Lombard Street from 1549 onwards and that he was not only a lender of money, but was also paying interest on deposits.

In the Middle Ages, the lending of money at interest rates was considered to be unChristian and was forbidden to Englishmen, some of whom were hanged for the offence. The taking of interest was stigmatized with usury on the strict interpretation of the law 'thou shal't not lend upon usury to thou brother'. The usury laws were partly abolished by Henry VIII in 1545, and the taking of interest on loans became legal; the rate was fixed at 10% per annum. In 1900, the Money Lenders' Act was passed and provided that if interest on a loan exceeded 48% per annum it must be presumed excessive!

The career of a GP will undergo many changes during his working life, from a trainee doctor to being, perhaps, a senior partner. At each stage in a career, different financial wants and needs will occur ranging from a junior doctor wondering how he will repay accumulated student debts and other loans, through to buying a car, a first home, one's way into a practice, finishing with the senior partner perhaps considering retirement and the sale of his share in a partnership. In everything concerning banking and financial affairs, the banker should be a centre of advice, support and direction without upsetting existing professional connections. It is not, however, always clear what banks offer or are able to do. An executive of Westpac, the Australian bank, has commented that 'by and large, banking products and services vary little between one bank and another . . . A bank must develop ways of delivering products and services that are tailor-made for customer needs and offer a return to the personalized service of the past'.

Although the basic principles of banking remain the same, enormous and far-reaching changes have taken place and continue to do so at an increasing rate. However, GPs should receive from their banker a first class banking service, delivered in an efficient, courteous and professional manner. Banks are a service industry and, although accountable to their owners, the shareholders, they must not lose sight of their customers who are the lifeblood of the business.

A GP has a right to expect from the bank a close working relationship and this can come about only by an understanding of the GP's needs. A bank should be able to advise and suggest ways in which a practitioner's banking arrangements could better be served. The needs for an efficient money transmission system are apparent, but the systems available from banks, or by contract with computer agencies, for the payment of staff salaries at almost no cost to the practitioner are less well known.

There will be occasions when the practice enjoys a surplus of funds when interest-bearing accounts, whilst still retaining ready access to the monies, will be of benefit. Conversely, there may be an occasional need for short-term borrowing facilities to meet the practitioner's cash flow requirements, or longer-term loans for items of equipment, computer systems and surgery development finance. In all these matters, a close working relationship will bring mutual benefits to both GP and banker and will allow the accounts to operate smoothly.

In the event that a practitioner becomes a fundholder, there will be additional needs to ensure that the monies passing through the account are used to the best benefit of the customer, and almost all banks now provide facilities whereby funds can be moved automatically between a current account and an interest-bearing account to ensure that the surplus funds are earning interest and to cover any overdrafts that may appear on the former. Some banks will even offer an interest-bearing business current account so that interest is earned automatically without having to move the money.

As a partnership is made up of individuals, apart from the joint and several liability that exists for any partnership debt, in discussing lending facilities, a banker should be aware of the individual's circumstances to ensure that any group decision about long-term finance will not be to the detriment of the individual. In essence, the banker should be acquainted with the GP's accountant and other professional advisers, to ensure that the advice given to the practitioner is based on due consideration of all the facts.

The competition for good quality banking business provides the GP with an array of choices and it is important for both bank and customer that a long-term, mutually trustful and respectful relationship is established, both with the practitioner and with the practice manager. GPs should consider which bank to use and take the opportunity to investigate what banking services each is able to offer. As a last resort, GPs can always move the account, and a personal recommendation to an efficient and effective manager is often the best source of introduction.

51 The GP and his Solicitor

Question: 'What have you got when a lawyer is buried up to his neck in the sand?'

Answer: 'Not enough sand.'

'What is black and brown and looks good on a lawyer?'
'A dobermann pinscher.'

'Why do they bury lawyers 12 feet under?'
'Because deep down they are good people.'

This is an important book. I feel free to say so because, apart from the jokes (which I cannot claim to have invented) and the rest of this chapter, I have not written any of it. What it contains is of great value to the GP and it has the merit of being clearly and succinctly presented so that busy people can readily understand and assimilate it.

There is, however, a danger in this for the unwary and the overconfident. A number of the topics which are covered do not give themselves readily to DIY. It is plain from the tone of such chapters that this is the case and that experts should be consulted. Depending on the circumstance, the expert might be:

- LMC secretary/chairman
- FHSA general manager
- BMA industrial relations officer
- practice banker
- practice accountant
- **solicitor.**

Solicitors specialize in a number of subjects covered in this book, including:

- employing staff (Chapter 15)
- partnership deeds (Chapter 22)
- the ownership of surgeries (Chapter 27)
- the cost rent scheme (Chapter 28).

The last of these topics is specialized in the particular sense that a solicitor who advises on it is likely to act regularly for GPs, advising them about the acquisition of new practice premises or the adaptation of existing ones. The concept of specialist solicitors is covered in more detail later in this chapter.

All good solicitors' firms have members who know about the laws of employment, partnership and real estate, and have practical experience of their application. Wherever a GP practises, there will almost certainly be such a firm nearby.

Is a partnership solicitor necessary?

The average practice is unlikely to need the services of a partnership solicitor to the extent that it needs those of the partnership accountant, whose role is described in Chapter 49 as a day-by-day hands-on role. It is to be hoped that there is no need for such intensive care from a solicitor.

However, an established relationship with the partnership solicitor is valuable. It is a question of habit and of testing possible courses of action on the solicitor before committing the practice to them.

For instance, if you are thinking of dismissing an employee for gross misconduct, pick up the telephone and take advice from your solicitor. You will learn immediately whether an industrial tribunal is likely to agree with you that the alleged misconduct warrants instant dismissal and, if not, the level of compensation the tribunal would order you to pay for unfair dismissal. On this basis, you and your partners will be able to decide on appropriate action.

Fees

Whereas the jokes at the beginning of this chapter are on lawyers, you may feel that, when it comes to legal fees, the joke is on you. However, a realistic solicitor will discuss with his clients, and potential clients, various methods of fixing fees. Hourly rates are the norm, but the concept of the proper rate for the job is making a welcome return to the field. Rules of professional practice now require advance warning of the likely fees.

A firm which anticipates being retained by a GP partnership, to give advice regularly on a variety of issues in which its members have experience, may be willing to negotiate an annual retainer.

The specialist solicitor

Some solicitors' firms specialize in issues such as the cost rent scheme, partnership deeds and partnership disputes, which are of vital importance to GPs. These firms may be approached for advice on individual issues, or they may be retained, on the GP's instructions, by the partnership solicitor when their specialist knowledge needs to be tapped. This has the advantage that the partnership solicitor need not be abandoned at the time when advice is needed most. These are called agency instructions and they work particularly well on partnership deeds, Red Book questions and highly specialized elements of premises acquisition and development.

The specialist firm will charge for its expertise, but remember that a specialist solicitor will spend significantly less chargeable hours on the job than one who has to research your particular problem virtually from scratch.

This chapter was contributed by Nick Gild, who is a solicitor.

52 Practice Meetings

SOME medical partnerships operate as such only financially, dividing profits on an agreed basis; although there may be a partnership deed, the partners appear to work as individual units. The partners never meet to discuss common policy, with the result that the practice is fractionalized and cannot work as a cohesive unit.

To ensure cohesion in the practice, partners should hold regular and systematic partnership meetings, where controversial matters can be discussed, decisions made and a policy determined. The most effective and well-organized partnerships are invariably those that work as a single unit, where the partners have a common policy and are aware of working towards a common goal. In recent years, this has in some cases been enshrined in a formal business plan (*see* Chapter 14).

Who should attend?

It is usually beneficial not to restrict attendance of practice meetings to the partners, but also to include trusted advisers and, in suitable cases, senior staff. The practice manager should also attend in an advisory capacity and in many training practices the current trainee also attends. Matters discussed at the meeting should be entirely confidential and those attending should be aware that this is the case.

There will be times, when special matters are discussed, that outside advice might be needed. For instance, if the partnership deed is to be considered, the solicitor may be invited to attend. If the practice accounts have recently been completed, the accountant may be asked to run through them prior to approval by the partners, and the architect may be asked to attend if a surgery development scheme is pending.

Timing

Regular dates throughout the year should be set aside for these meetings (for instance, the second Tuesday in each month at 7.30 pm). The exact timing will depend on the conditions applying in the particular practice: some practices find it more convenient to hold meetings after surgery hours; others prefer them to be held during the lunch break. In any event, it is essential that adequate notice be given so that diaries may be organized and appointments made accordingly.

Agendas

An agenda should be circulated at least a week before the meeting and partners should be invited to place items on the agenda for discussion. It is important that any item of a controversial and difficult nature is included in the agenda, and not raised under 'any other business' so that those attending may consider the matter beforehand. Indeed, any matter under AOB, unless it is of abiding urgency, should be held over until the next meeting.

A typical agenda for a practice meeting is set out in Figure 52.1. This is normally prepared by the practice manager.

THE BRANCASTER GROUP PRACTICE

Practice Meeting: Tuesday 13 July 1993
To be held in the Common Room: 7.30 pm

AGENDA

1. To confirm the minutes of the meeting held on 15 June 1993 (previously circulated).
2. Matters arising from the meeting.
3. Clinical matters (Dr Black).
4. Executive partner's report (Dr White):

    4.1 Financial position
    4.2 Bank loan
    4.3 New 1993/94 drawings figures
    4.4 New income tax reserves
    4.5 Arrangement for June 1993 accounts.

5. Practice manager's report (Mrs Grey):

    5.1 Staffing levels
    5.2 Ancillary staff refund
    5.3 Rota.

6. New partnership agreement (Mr Deedes, practice solicitor, will attend).
7. Surgery extension project (Dr Brown):

    7.1 FHSA agreement
    7.2 Building contract
    7.3 Bridging finance
    7.4 Architect's report.

8. Any other business.
9. Next meeting (17 August).

Figure 52.1   A typical agenda for a practice meeting

Minutes

Minutes should be taken by someone delegated by the partners for that purpose, usually the practice manager although it may be suitable for a confidential secretary to attend for that purpose.

Chairman

It is necessary to appoint a chairman for each meeting. Some partnerships prefer the senior partner to take the chair at every meeting and he would normally expect to do so. Others find it preferable for the chair to 'rotate', with a different person taking the chair at each meeting on a rota basis. This system is also useful for introducing younger partners to the problems of leadership and may allow them to see the problems of the practice in a different light.

In larger partnerships, it is normal to delegate aspects of practice management to certain of the partners. Each of these partners should report at practice meetings. For instance, there may be a partner in overall charge of finances, one responsible for the surgery building, another for staff, one for training, and so on.

Duration of meetings

It is usually a good idea to fix a maximum amount of time for each meeting. This not only encourages attendance but it enables the chairman to allocate time for discussion of each item without allowing it to drag on unduly.

Appendix A:
Fees and Allowances for GPs, 1994/95

		From 1 April 1994 to 31 March 1995 £

Practice allowances

Maximum for:	BPA: full rate	6816
Designated area:	Type I	3315
	Type II	5055
Seniority:	Stage I	425
	Stage II	2215
	Stage III	4770
Postgraduate education allowance (full rate)		2150
Trainee supervison grant		4675
Assistant's allowance:	Ordinary	5925
	In designated area	8295
Associate allowance* (max: 3rd year)		25 675
Leave advance (20% of BPA)		1363

Capitation fees

Standard		
Age:	To 64	14.60
	65–74	19.30
	75 and over	37.30
Addition for out-of-hours		2.90
Deprivation payments:	High level	10.20
(per patient)	Medium level	7.65
	Low level	5.85
New registration		6.45
Child health surveillance		10.60
Rural practice: unit payment		0.219

Target payments (maximum per doctor)

Childhood immunizations: Higher		2145
Lower		715

		£
Pre-school boosters:	Higher	630
	Lower	210
Cervical cytology:	Higher	2415
	Lower	805

Sessional payments

Health promotion clinics		
Per Band (annual fee)		
	Band 1	430.00
	Band 2	1160.00
	Asthma and diabetes	
	care (each)	360.00 (× 2)
	Band 3	2060.00
Minor surgery		106.20
Teaching medical students		12.00

Item of service fees, etc

Night visit fee:	Higher	47.85
	Lower	15.95
Maternity fees** (obst list: complete service)		169.00

Fees per patient

Anaesthetic fee		35.80
IUCD		46.35
Contraception		13.55
Emergency treatment and minor ops*		21.45
Temporary resident:	To 15 days	8.60
	Over 15 days	12.90
Vaccination:	Lower	5.15
	Higher	3.55
Dental haemorrhage:	Higher	21.45
	Lower	14.60

Locum allowance in sickness (weekly maximum)	405.60

*   Please refer to detailed fees as published from time to time.
** A full scale of maternity fees, depending on whether or not the doctor is on
     the obstetric list, is available from most medical journals.

More complete details and updated information on current rates of fees
and allowances can be obtained monthly from the main medical journals:
Medeconomics, *Financial Pulse* and *Money Pulse*.

Appendix B:
Income Tax Rates and Personal
Allowances, 1994/95 and 1995/96

Income tax rates

The basic and higher rates bands for 1994/95 are as follows.

1994/95:

Taxable income	Rate of tax	Band	Tax on band
£	%	£	£
0–3000	20	3000	600
3001–23 700	25	20 700	5175
23 701 and over	40	–	–

1995/96:

0–3200	20	3200	640
3201–24 300	25	21 100	5275
24 301 and over	40	–	–

Personal allowances

	1995/96 £	1994/95 £
Single person's allowance	3525	3445
Married couple's allowance*	1720	1720
Age allowance (single): 65–74	4630	4200
Over 74	4800	4370
Age allowance (married): 65–74	2995	2665
Over 74	3035	2705
Income limit for age allowance	14 600	14 200
Allowance for single parent families*	1720	1720
*Relief limited to:	15%	20%

Capital gains tax

	1995/96	1994/95
Annual exemption limit	6000	5800
Rate of charge	At income tax rates	At income tax rates
Retirement relief:		
Exempt gain	150 000	150 000

(Plus on half the gain between £150 000 and £600 000)

Appendix C:
National Insurance Rates, 1994/95 and 1995/96

Class 1: Percentage of weekly wage/salary (not contracted out)

	Employee %	Employer %
1994/95:		
To £56.99	Nil	Nil
£57–99.99 ⎫	2% of £57 and	3.61
£100–144.99 ⎬	10% on remainder	5.62
£145–199.99 ⎭	up to £430	7.68
From £200		10.2
1995/96:		
To £58.99	Nil	Nil
£59–104.99 ⎫	2% of £59 and	3
£105–149.99 ⎬	10% on remainder	5
£150–204.99 ⎭	up to £440	7
From £205		10.2

	1995/96 £	1994/95 £
Class 2: Self-employed (flat-rate) contributions		
Weekly (by direct debit or quarterly charge)	5.85	5.65
Small earnings exemption threshold	3310	3200
Class 3: Non-employed contributions		
Weekly stamp	5.75	5.55
Class 4: Self-employed (earnings-related) contributions		
Lower income threshold	6640	6490
Upper income threshold	22 880	22 360
Rate charged	7.3%	7.3%
Maximum contribution (pa)	1185.52	1158.51

Appendix D:
Tax Relief on Pension Contributions

Inland Revenue extra-statutory concession on doctors' and dentists' superannuation contributions

The following is an extract from the Regulations.

Under FA 1970, s 22 (for 1973/74 onwards; ICTA 1970, s 209 for years to 1972/73) contributions required to be made in pursuance of a public general Act of Parliament by the holder of an office or employment towards the provisions of superannuation benefits may be deducted in assessing his emoluments. These sections are in practice treated as extending to assessments under Schedule D on the profits of a medical or dental practitioner who is required to make superannuation contributions in pursuance of the National Health Service Acts. Where, however, the practitioner also pays premiums or contributions towards a retirement annuity within ICTA 1970, s 226 a restriction is imposed either on the amount of the deduction for his statutory contribution or on the amount of retirement annuity relief allowable.

For 1980/81 onwards concessionary relief is allowable on either of the following bases.

Either practitioners may have relief on the amount of their NHS contributions together with relief on the amount of any retirement annuity premium in relation to their non-NHS earnings. For this purpose:

(i)   non-NHS earnings are taken as the amount of net relevant earnings (as defined in Sec 227(5)) less the sum produced by multiplying the amount of the NHS contributions by 16⅓.
(ii) retirement annuity relief will be allowable within the normal limit of 17½% (or the higher percentages for older contributors) of the non-NHS earnings plus any unused relief for earlier years. For this purpose unused relief should be calculated on the appropriate concessional basis for years in which relief has been allowed on NHS contributions.

Or, practitioners may have relief on the same basis as set out in 2 relating to the years 1972/73 to 1979/80.*

Finally, practitioners may, instead, have relief on a statutory basis. In this case, they would take retirement annuity relief, up to the limits appropriate for a particular year, on their full net relevant earnings (ie including NHS earnings). But in that event no concessionary relief would be available in respect of NHS contributions.

Source   IRI (1970) as amended and updated by each of the Supplements 1971 to 1975: 1977 and 1978 Supplements to IRI (1976) and amended to present wording by 1981 Supplement to IRI (1980).

Notes   In view of the number of changes that have been made to this concession (see sources above), careful consideration should be given to the exact form of the concession for earlier years.

*2   Alternatively, practitioners may have relief on the amount of their NHS contributions together with relief on any retirement annuity premiums paid up to the amount of the largest premium on which tax relief was allowed for any of the three years 1969/70 to 1971/72— but with a restriction, if necessary, to keep the total relief on NHS contributions and retirement annuity premiums within the pre-1971/ 72 limits for retirement annuity relief at 10% of net relevant earnings or £730—or the higher limits permitted to older people. Any surplus of premiums paid over the amount allowable on this basis will not be available for carry-forward.

   The Finance Act 1980 removed the ceilings on premiums payable and introduced carry-forward.

Appendix E:
Area Bands for Cost Rent Limits:
building cost location factors

FHSA	£
England	
Avon	0.94
Barking and Havering	1.07
Barnet	1.07
Barnsley	0.96
Bedfordshire	1.00
Berkshire	1.01
Birmingham	0.94
Bolton	1.03
Bradford	0.93
Brent and Harrow	1.14
Bromley	1.07
Buckinghamshire	1.01
Bury	1.03
Calderdale	0.92
Cambridgeshire	1.01
Camden and Islington	1.14
Cheshire	1.01
City and E. London	1.14
Cleveland	0.93
Cornwall and Isles of Scilly	0.90
Coventry	0.94
Croydon	1.07
Cumbria	1.02
Derbyshire	0.92
Devon	0.90
Doncaster	0.96
Dorset	0.97
Dudley	0.94
Durham	0.94
Ealing, Hammersmith and Hounslow	1.14

East Sussex	1.06
Enfield and Haringey	1.07
Essex	0.99
Gateshead	0.97
Gloucestershire	0.92
Greenwich and Bexley	1.14
Hampshire	0.97
Hereford and Worcester	0.92
Hertfordshire	1.07
Hillingdon	1.07
Humberside	1.00
Isle of Wight	0.93
Kensington, Chelsea and Westminster	1.14
Kent	1.05
Kingston and Richmond	1.07
Kirklees	0.93
Lambeth, Southwark and Lewisham	1.14
Lancashire	1.04
Leeds	0.93
Leicestershire	0.95
Lincolnshire	0.92
Liverpool	1.03
Manchester	1.03
Merton, Sutton and Wandsworth	1.07
Newcastle	0.97
Norfolk	0.96
Northamptonshire	0.90
North Tyneside	0.97
Northumberland	1.00
North Yorkshire	0.99
Nottinghamshire	0.93
Oldham	1.03
Oxfordshire	0.97
Redbridge and Waltham Forest	1.07
Rochdale	1.03
Rotherham	0.96
St Helens and Knowsley	1.03
Salford	1.03
Sandwell	0.94
Sefton	1.03
Sheffield	0.96

Shropshire	0.91
Solihull	0.94
Somerset	0.91
South Tyneside	0.97
Staffordshire	0.91
Stockport	1.03
Suffolk	1.00
Sunderland	1.47
Surrey	1.10
Tameside	1.03
Trafford	1.03
Wakefield	0.92
Walsall	0.94
Warwickshire	0.98
West Sussex	1.02
Wigan	1.03
Wiltshire	0.94
Wirral	1.03
Wolverhampton	0.94

Wales

Clwyd	0.98
Dyfed	0.96
Mid Glamorgan	0.96
South Glamorgan	0.98
West Glamorgan	0.93
Gwent	0.96
Gwynedd	0.93
Powys	0.91

Appendix F:
Current Cost Rent Limits

Building cost limits per practice unit:	From May 1993 Rate A* £	Rate B** £
One GP	40 414	35 126
Two GPs	73 954	64 285
Three GPs	111 196	96 767
Four GPs	135 142	117 541
Five GPs	159 617	138 767
Six GPs	180 088	156 596
Seven GPs	202 751	176 311
Eight GPs	225 111	195 724
Nine GPs	247 773	215 441

Optional extra rooms:

offices per m^2	370	320
common room per m^2	370	320
dispensary per m^2	370	320
plus externals	15%	15%
plus professional fees	11.5%	11.5%
with VAT	17.5%	17.5%
plus planning consent fees	100%	100%
plus approved site cost	100%	100%

All costs exclude VAT, which will be added by the FHSA at the rate currently in force.

* For new developments and approved works, plus VAT.
** For modifications of existing buildings, plus VAT.

Index